Clinics in Developmental Medicine No. 112

DEVELOPMENTAL EXAMINATION OF INFANTS AND PRESCHOOL CHILDREN

DOROTHY F. EGAN

Formerly Honorary Consultant Paediatrician,
Newcomen Centre, Guy's Hospital, St Thomas St., London

1990
Mac Keith Press
OXFORD: Blackwell Scientific Publications Ltd.
PHILADELPHIA: J. B. Lippincott Co.

5a Netherhall Gardens, London NW3 5RN

First published 1990

British Library Cataloguing in Publication Data

Egan, Dorothy F.
Developmental examination of infants and preschool children
1. Children. Growth. Assessment
I. Title II. Series
612.65

ISBN (UK) 0-632-02846-7
(USA) 0-397-48022-9

Printed in Great Britain at The Lavenham Press Ltd., Lavenham, Suffolk
Mac Keith Press is supported by **The Spastics Society, London, England**

To Bill with love

CONTENTS

FOREWORD

It is a very great pleasure to see Dorothy Egan's book complete and to have the privilege of introducing it. It contains the distilled wisdom of a lifetime spent observing, assessing and enjoying the company of young children. It is worth saying at the outset that Dorothy has been the outstanding clinician and teacher in the field of early child development in the UK for the past 20 years.

The 'test bed' for the subject was a remarkable group of people who were assembled by Ronnie Mac Keith at Guy's from the late 1950s and included Mary Sheridan, Dorothy Egan, Jessie Francis-Williams, David Scrutton, Molly Playfair, Peter Robson and Martin Bax. Mary produced the basic tests and the team, particularly Dorothy, used and developed them. They did pioneering work on the comprehensive assessment and care of disabled children, goal-orientated community therapy and the integration of hospital and community services for children with neurological disability. Several surgeons were keen to be part of this new approach. The team developed working relationships with their regional colleagues and were eventually seeing several thousand children annually. A typical assessment took 1½ hours and involved two or three people. By the time the paediatric neurologists joined, we were happy and grateful to use this form of combined assessment. As a result, the neurological diagnosis which followed the assembling of a developmental problem list became more secure; and in the process of finding treatable and genetic diseases and conditions with a characteristic natural history, we would not be without this dimension to the clinical examination. Of particular value is the carefully documented performance of a child in whom the diagnosis is not clear at the initial visit.

The story behind the standardisation of the tests is worth telling. Dorothy Egan had been using these methods, modifying them in the light of experience, and teaching them to hundreds of doctors. Her pupils were usually surprised at what children would do if you were able to encourage them appropriately, and felt that their paediatric perspective had been widened. These assessments were not intended to give precise developmental ages, but to indicate which children needed further investigation and help. When it was pointed out that accumulated experience was not the same as a population-based study, Dorothy retired from active clinical practice at the age of 80 and set about this essential and extensive piece of research. Although there were few surprises, significant modifications of the tests did come out of these studies of the performance of normal children.

Dr Egan presents child development as a story in which learning is the product of innate ability, practice, and parental encouragement. She allows you to make up your own mind about their relative importance. Her analysis of the learning process encourages the examiner to do more than just 'test' the child. The child's interest and drive is recognised, engaged, responded to and respected. The point is not that a child learns manual release, for instance, by throwing forwards rather than by observation, but that this is the simplest explanation of the observed sequence. It gives the examiner additional clues which link one developmental stage to the next, and introduces the idea of quality and style of performance. These aspects and the subject of attention control are not pursued in detail.

This book is relevant to modern paediatric practice. It adds an important clinical skill to paediatricians and others who need to assess young children, and it could be seen as a basic requirement. It encourages us to make a direct relationship with young children and to develop our observational skills. Parents are helped by seeing that their child has 'performed' and that medical decisions in the area of development are made on the basis of objective evidence as well as that given in the history. With the increasing technical complexity of modern paediatrics it is essential that those caring for very sick children have a personal level of skill in the assessment of cognitive and special sensory function. The ethical decisions that face professionals and parents are difficult enough, even with all the relevant data. Brain imaging is not a substitute for clinical examination.

This book will complement the usual method of acquiring these skills, which is a short course of lectures, demonstrations and tutored practice. The developmental examination is neither a screening test nor the last word in the detailed analysis of any particular area of development. It provides a quick method of looking at a child who may have a problem. Normal results are very reassuring. Abnormal results lead to further detailed, including neurological, investigation.

Here, therefore, is the definitive account of a scheme of developmental assessment which developed in the UK but which is of wide application and will continue to exert a strong influence on paediatrics.

BRIAN NEVILLE,
Professor of Paediatric Neurology,
Institute of Child Health,
Guilford Street, London.

PREFACE

Paediatricians in the United Kingdom became interested in developmental paediatrics through the efforts of a few individuals. Gesell's classic studies were interpreted for them by Ronald Illingworth, among others, and Mary Sheridan's pioneering work gave new insights into the developmental problems of young children. Then in the 1960s a paediatrician at Guy's Hospital, Ronald Mac Keith, started to play an increasingly important role. As director of the Spastics Society's Medical Education and Information Unit he proved to have a special ability to stimulate and facilitate discussion and enquiry. In 1964 he set up the Newcomen Child Development Centre for disabled children at Guy's, and was later joined there by Mary Sheridan and myself.

The Centre began its work in a disused Victorian pub just outside the back gate of the hospital. Consulting rooms, never designed for the purpose, had a friendly and lived-in atmosphere. The steep winding stair, up which disabled children were carried (or climbed with dogged determination), in no way curbed the enthusiasm of the staff or, more importantly, of parents. Eventually the building became too small and the Centre was moved into a vacant neighbouring school, and next into portakabins at the foot of Guy's Tower, where the paediatric wards had recently been opened. Here the Centre remained and here Ronnie, as he was affectionately known, led his team until his retirement in 1974. He was and remains an inspiration to us all.

Thirteen years were to pass before Brian Neville, who then became Director of the Centre, was able to move his team into a splendid purpose-built unit.

Increasing recognition has been given to its achievements in the care of disabled children, in its research into methods to help them to achieve new skills, and in its training courses in developmental paediatrics for hospital doctors, general practitioners and child health doctors. During the years I was privileged to work as a member of the team, all too often we were moved by the distress of parents, who, having consulted various professional advisers on some aspect of their child's development which worried them, had been reassured with the words: 'He will grow out of it'. It seemed to me then that what was needed was a practical guide to a simple developmental examination using standardised tests that can reveal those children whose development is proceeding within normal limits and those who warrant further investigation.

My grateful thanks go to Dr Anthony Golding and Dr John Meadows who gave facilities for clinical research, to their health visitors, and to the several practitioners who generously allowed me to see children in their busy practices.

I am enormously indebted to Brian Neville who gave me the opportunity to continue my work with disabled children and to teach these skills, and who encouraged me to write this book.

My thanks, too, to all my loyal family and, in particular, to Tricie for valuable help and guidance, and to Bill who urged me on.

February 1990 DOROTHY F. EGAN

INTRODUCTION

This book is a practical guide to general practitioners, child health doctors and health visitors* engaged in the promotion of health and welfare of young children. Its concern is to reveal a developmental problem which may cause learning difficulties in early childhood. The age-range is from six weeks to 4½ years. The tests described may also be useful for older children functioning within this age-range.

Infants at risk of severe disability arising from pre- or perinatal conditions are today commonly diagnosed in the neonatal period and followed up by hospital paediatricians. Some with impairments may be missed and will be brought in the first instance to the general practitioner or child health doctor. Less severe deficits may be hidden and delay development in the early childhood years.

Great changes have occurred in our thinking in the last 25 years, following the introduction of clinical tests of hearing in the first year of life in child health centres; training courses in developmental 'screening' for child health doctors; health education programmes; and the emergence of the neonatologist, and the setting up of child development centres. With today's advances in developmental procedures, we can at least identify some problems that may cause learning difficulties.

Parents are often the first to suspect that something is amiss. How many children may have been wrongly diagnosed because we did not know how to decide whether they could hear, see or understand?

The general practitioner must decide whether to set up a formal scheme in the practice, for developmental examination of children under five years of age. All those responsible for the medical care of young children will sometimes need to use such procedures. A deficit occurring in any of the pathways of development (vision, hearing, language, performance skills, intellect or gross motor development) can not only affect progress in the relevant area, but may also modify the whole pattern.

The learning process begins at birth, and parents have a vital role to play in

**General practitioners,* often referred to as family doctors, provide general medical care at a local level, or when necessary by referral to hospital specialists and others. Some may conduct child health clinics for children on their medical list.

Child health doctors work in community health centres with a team of health visitors. They have a preventative role in advising mothers (within a designated area) on the health of infants and preschool children; in carrying out immunisation programmes, and in offering developmental examinations at several crucial stages in the first five years. Referral for medical treatment is made through the child's own general practitioner. Child health doctors are also part of the primary health-care team which includes health visitors, therapists and the community paediatrician.

Health visitors are qualified nurses who have undertaken further training. They are part of the primary health-care team, and usually work from a health centre or family doctor's group practice. Their duty is to visit all newborn babies a few weeks after birth, and to help and instruct mothers in all aspects of child care, including feeding and immunisations. They have a particular responsibility to assist, advise and provide contact for parents of children with a disability or special needs or problems.

their child's development. Lack of parental attention in the formative years may seriously affect the developmental progress a child is likely to make. Attaining the full intellectual potential is important not just to the individual child, but also to the community in which he lives.

Normal development follows the complex interaction of several pathways of development which are summarised in this book. An infant's first steps in new phases of learning are expected to emerge at known age-levels. These are listed for easy reference at the end of each of three stages of development.

The 'craft' of developmental examination includes hints on making and maintaining a social relationship with a young child, while encouraging him to give of his best under experimental conditions. If certain principles are understood and used, the task may prove less daunting.

The objective of this book is to present simple and quick tests which doctors and health visitors can use to reveal a developmental problem. A developmental examination is in two parts—first a careful history of pregnancy, labour and the puerperium, the child's development to date, family history of disability and the parents' own view of their child's development; second, tests of development to reveal substantial low scores in language and/or performance skills, defects of hearing and vision, and delay in gross motor development. The results must be considered in the light of any abnormal physical findings, or disorders known to affect development adversely. Details of physical examination are not included in this book.

The techniques of developmental examination described have been used by the author over a period of some 20 years at the Newcomen Child Development Centre, Guy's Hospital, for children with severe disabling conditions as well as more mild deficits. Norms for children between six weeks and 20 months are based on Gesell scales using tests previously described by Sheridan (1975, 1976), some of which have been updated and standardised. Patterns of procedures appropriate to each of three stages of development are presented.

A developmental examination of children from 20 months to 4½ years (including a language/performance profile, and vision and hearing tests) has been standardised by the author on a sample of 425 children living in an inner-city area or a rural market town. 30 per cent of the sample consisted of children from ethnic minorities.

My test of developing language and performance skills (Egan bus puzzle test, see page 56), assesses comprehension and expressive language separately, and provides a data base in graphical form with which to compare an individual child's variation from the average and to calculate his age-level equivalent. Performance skills in copying cube models, geometric shapes, and the draw-a-man test have also been standardised. Graphs are provided, to show when delay might be suspected.

A developmental examination at primary-care level is not about diagnosis of a particular disorder; it is about distinguishing between those whose development is proceeding within normal limits, and those who warrant further investigation. The normative graphs presented in our scheme permit this by revealing the lowest 20 per cent as well as the average.

The kind of action to be taken depends on the judgement of the doctor, and the probable co-operation of parents themselves, as well as the availability of local services to establish a diagnosis and to provide therapy and helpful training.

The miniature toy test for language development, first designed as an unstandardised free-play situation (Sheridan 1975), is less suited to the needs of child health doctors and general practitioners. The actions of young children in this situation are often ambiguous and difficult to interpret. The test is more suited to the skills of secondary-care paediatricians. A standardised version of the test is included.

I have used the pronoun 'he' throughout the text to designate a child of either sex. I feel that the constant use of 'he or she' becomes tedious for the reader. Where any difference in behaviour of boys and girls has occurred, this is made clear in the text.

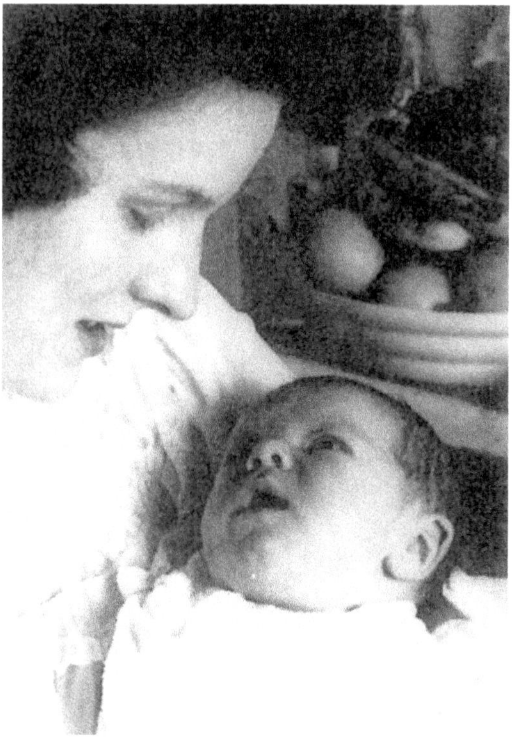

Frontispiece. Social communication: eye-to-eye contact within two hours of birth.

1
NORMAL DEVELOPMENT

A baby has an innate will to achieve, which is fostered initially by social communication with the mother. The reward of her smiles and affectionate gestures stimulates a baby to repeat his action, and thus initiates the first step to a new phase of learning. An infant finds pleasure in repetition and acquires a sense of his own ability. Once a skill has been mastered, interest rapidly fades as fresh drives take its place and lead to increasing dexterity and fine manipulation, gradual understanding of gestures and situations, and to the formation of concepts.

A newborn baby opens his eyes to a world of movement and shapes among which the human face becomes his major interest. Progress is broadly determined by maturation in the central nervous system, and is influenced by a number of major factors. First, there is a complex interaction of the several pathways of development: vision, hearing, language, performance skills, gross motor development and intellect. A deficit in any one pathway may adversely affect development in others, and a severe deficit may change the whole pattern of a child's development. Second, a baby's innate 'drive'—interest in his environment and will to master it—influences his progress through repeated practice of learned skills. It is hard work being a baby. At six months he can co-ordinate his hand movements to pick up a small toy on the table, and will practise until he can pick up two. Once he can use a superior pincer grasp to pick up a toy, at 10 months, an infant throws forward until release from his hand is competent. A series of permanent changes is thus established.

Third, experience of a wide variety of activities, and of social and mental interaction with adults and later with other children, is necessary in the first five years to enhance a child's potential. Play begins as an integral part of communication between mother and child. Without this interchange, progress can be seriously jeopardised. An extreme example of the adverse effects of severe early deprivation was seen in the early 1950s when illegitimate babies were often cared for in residential nurseries. Infants in the first nine months spent the day isolated in a cot—a precaution against the spread of gastro-enteritis which was rife in such institutions. Interaction with an adult was limited to periods of feeding and changing by a nurse who had several other babies yet to be fed and toileted. Proffered a brightly coloured toy by a friendly visitor, a six- to seven-month-old brought up in these circumstances might raise his hands, fingers spread wide, until they retreated behind his head and with a look of fear on his face utterly reject a situation he had not learned to understand. This is in marked contrast to the outgoing friendly response to strangers shown by a normal baby of this age.

Normal development is a continuum passing through a number of well defined stages, each of which is characterised by the appearance and maturing of definitive skills.

TABLE 1.I

Important developmental stages: six weeks to six months

Average age	*Vision*	*Hearing*	*Motor*	*Social communication*
Birth	Pupils react	Startles to sound	Primitive responses	Eye-to-eye contact
6 weeks	Visual fixation and following	Sounds at 15cm—stilling and eye-widening Recognises mother's voice	Head support in upright posture, 3 sec	Smiling response
12 weeks	Controlled visual attention by finger play		Midline posture of head for most of time	Vocalisations — vowel sounds
16 weeks	Hand regard	Turns head to side from which sounds come	Reaches for suspended toy Primitive responses pass off	
18 weeks	Knee regard		Raises head from mattress	Two-way vocalisations
22 weeks	Sees waving feet Visual tracking of falling toy		Legs up in vertical Grasps ankle and takes foot to his mouth	Loud vocalisations and 'raspberries'

Development can usefully be studied in three stages: (i) six weeks to six months, (ii) six months to 20 months, and (iii) 20 months to 4½ years. The average age when important skills are expected to emerge is given in the text and listed in tabular form at the end of each section for easy reference. Some variation within certain limits is to be expected and it must be emphasised that there is a normal range of development. Developmental delay should be suspected when important skills fail to emerge by the expected upper age-limit. For example, the social smile appears on average at six weeks of age. If a baby is not smiling back at nine or 10 weeks there is something wrong. Allowance is made for preterm birth. Useful tests of developing skills are described in some detail (see Chapters 6, 7 and 8). The descriptions of the tests include the upper age-limit when infants in the first two stages should have developed important skills. Children in the third developmental stage, whose abilities in the language/performance profile fall into the lowest 20 per cent of the range, are identified as those having substantial developmental delay requiring further investigation.

Stage 1: six weeks to six months (Table 1.I)

Vision is the dominant modality, as it: (i) promotes social communication; (ii) stimulates touch, reach and grasp, and encourages spatial recognition; (iii) influences the development of balancing reactions; (iv) reinforces auditory learning, and (v) contributes to the acquisition of language.

A neonate at birth is able to see. His pupils react to light. Held upright and turned slowly round in a circle, his eyes turn towards diffuse light from a window. Social communication can be seen within hours of birth as eye-to-eye contact with mother. A young baby finds the human face and gratings more interesting to look at than plain images and this can be demonstrated soon after birth. Fleeting smiles are described by some mothers during the early weeks; they may represent a baby's initial attempt to imitate his mother's facial movements. Some babies definitely copy the way she protrudes her tongue or purses her lips at six weeks.

The social smile appears on average at six weeks. It is a dazzling experience to parents, and few mothers forget when it was first seen. His smile is engendered by her expression as she smiles and nods; by her voice as she speaks leaning down close to his face; by the light touch of her fingers on his face and chest, and probably also by her smell. Such interactions promote social awareness.

A neonate startles to a sudden noise but after a few weeks as household sounds become more familiar he shows less response. He appears to recognise his mother's voice as different from others and is clearly soothed by it. He makes soft vocalisations.

Ability to focus the eye for near vision is poorly developed in the early weeks but momentary convergence may be seen from the eighth week.

In the first weeks a baby lies with his head turned to one side. Primitive grasping with the fingers and toes is strong. Placing, support and stepping is induced when the baby is held upright with the dorsum of the foot under the edge of a table. These primitive responses fade from 14 to 16 weeks, and for the next few weeks a baby no longer takes weight fully on his feet.

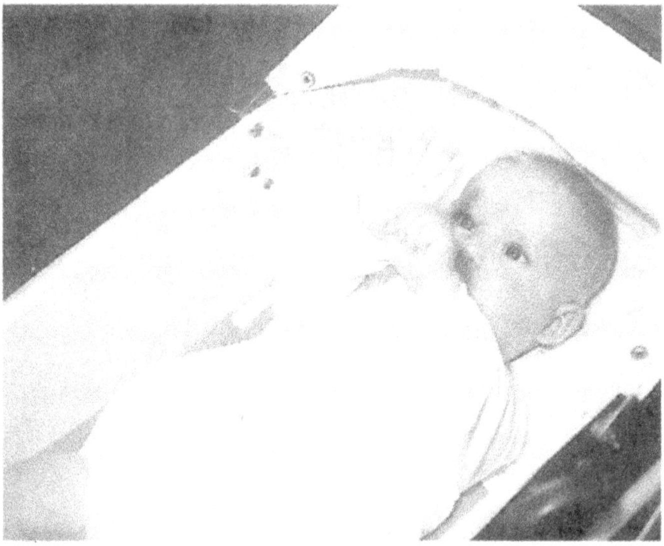

Fig. 1.1. Finger play at 14 wceks. Conscious control of visual function.

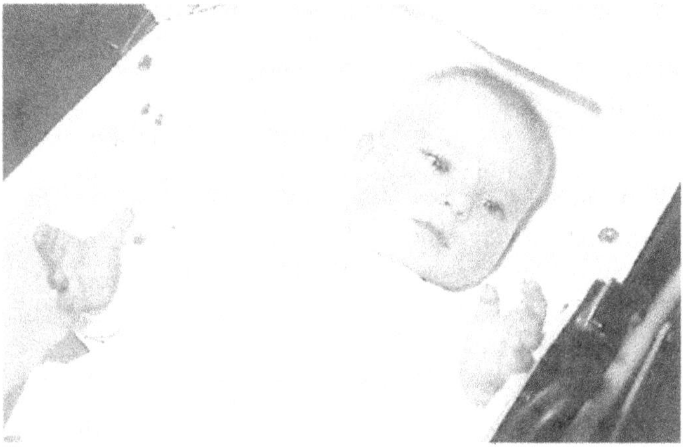

Fig. 1.2. Hand regard at 16 weeks.

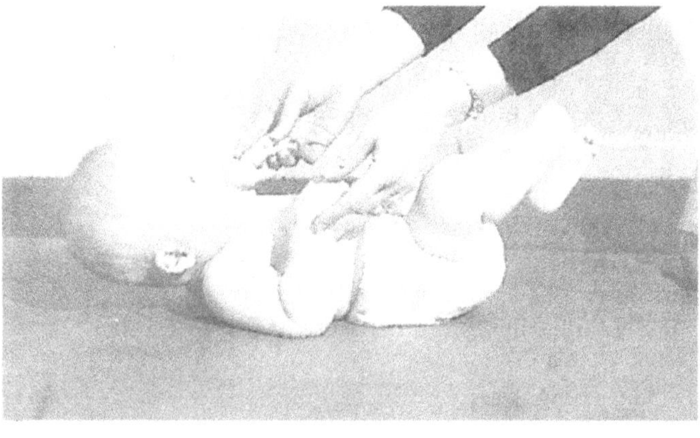

Fig. 1.3. Spontaneous lifting of the head at 18 weeks.

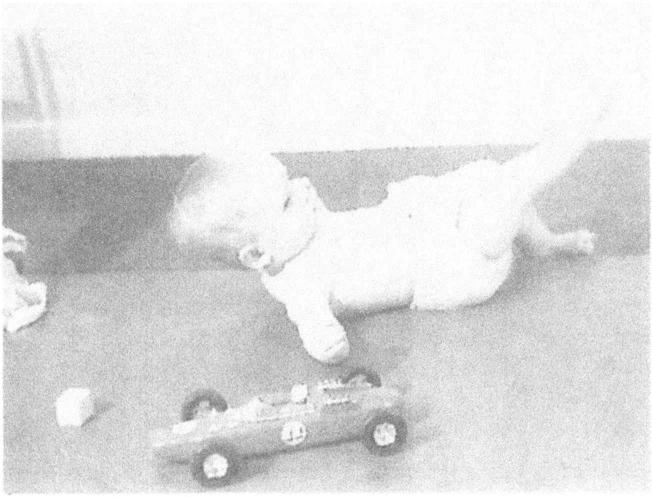

Fig. 1.4. Legs up in the vertical at 22 weeks.

A midline posture of the head is adopted for some 50 per cent of the time at 12 weeks. Concurrent changes in visual function enable a baby consciously to control visual attention at very near distance (Braddick 1986). He brings his fingers near to his face in order to inspect them closely and touches one finger with another to learn that they are part of himself (Fig. 1.1). Soon he begins to 'starfish' his fingers and converges his eyes to look at them. At 16 weeks he looks at his hands held at arm's length and begins to reach for a suspended or proffered toy (Fig. 1.2).

The ability to lift the head up from supine emerges at 18 weeks (Fig. 1.3). He cannot get up further unless mother pulls him up. As a baby practises this new skill he catches sight of his flexed knees and clutches his clothes in a determined effort to see more of these exciting objects.

By 16 weeks he shows interest in sounds three feet away from his ear and turns towards them, although as yet he is unable to locate their exact source. At 18 weeks he greets the appearance of mother's face over the side of his cot with a brilliant smile and excited movements of the limbs. He responds with tuneful vocalisations in turn with her when she speaks to him. In the next weeks he will readily respond to any friendly face and soft talk. This 'taking turns' is an essential component of communication.

Balancing reactions appear from the 16th week and progress may perhaps be stimulated in the following months by 'rough' play. A father may put his six-month-old daughter astride his shoulders and, holding her by one ankle, allow her to reach up for a balloon hanging from the ceiling. Balancing reactions can be demonstrated by holding a baby upright and tilting him sideways. Such passive movement in space stimulates proprioceptor and vestibular feedback, which is complemented by alteration in visual perception, so that the baby adjusts his head and thrusts out his arms and legs to restore his balance. Saving responses will appear in the next few weeks and complement balance.

A baby can actively extend the knee joint when the hip joint is flexed at the right angle, at 22 weeks, and his legs go up into the vertical (Fig. 1.4). The sight of

TABLE 1.II

Important developmental stages: seven to 20 months

				Language	
Average age	*Vision*	*Hearing*	*Performance*	*Comprehension*	*Expressive language*
7 months	Visual attention at 1m	Locates sound at 1m on ear level	Object permanence begins Palmar grasp Transfers		Double sounds
9–11 months	Visual attention at 3m	Locates sound at 1m above ear level	Inferior pincer grasp Superior pincer grasp Throws forward Releases from hand	Understands gesture and simple action words	Imitative babble
12 months				Pointing gesture	
13–15 months	Visual attention up to 6m		Finger release from 13 months	Self-related symbolic play with real objects	Jargons
15 months				Selects 3 or 4 objects from naming	
18 months			Builds at least 3 cubes	Detached-from-self symbolic play with real objects	Names 4–6 familiar objects or pictures
19–20 months			Beginning to recognise shapes	Understands names of up to 20 familiar objects	

Gross motor skills: sits unsupported at 6½–7 months. Crawls, pulls to stand, steps sideways and walks. This sequence of events is variable and depends on race, culture and family. Some 15 per cent of families do not have prone pattern of learning to walk.

his waving feet stimulates him to reach out and grasp his foot and thus discover that this too is part of himself. The baby's controlled visual attention has gradually extended through his own body, and he has learned something of the potential functional capacity of different parts of his motor system (arms for prehension and legs for mobility) (Sonksen *et al.* 1984).

A baby of 22 to 24 weeks, sitting supported on his mother's lap, shows an immediate interest in a small object on the table. He pats with his hands held flat and fingers spread wide in an eager attempt to reach it, but hand movements are as yet insufficiently co-ordinated for him to succeed. Some determined babies may duck the head with open mouth in an effort to get the desired object. Vocalisations now include loud sounds and blowing 'raspberries'.

The 5½-month-old baby watches a ball rolling across the table, and tracks it visually when it falls over the edge within his view. If it disappears over the table's outer edge, he instantly looks away and appears no longer to realise its existence.

Stage 2: seven months to 20 months (Table 1.II)

An infant of seven months reaches immediately for a cube on the table, patting with his hand held flat, to scoop it up in a palmar grasp using all his fingers but not the thumb. He immediately takes the cube to his mouth. During the next two weeks or so, holding it close to his mouth, he brings up the other hand and thus learns to transfer the cube from one hand to the other. By eight months he takes one in each hand and sometimes approaches with an extended index finger. An index finger approach is constant from nine months and the grasp becomes inferior pincer—terminal phalanx of index and second fingers with the thumb.

At six months an infant shows an immediate interest in meaningful sounds on his ear level and is impelled to turn and locate the source, though he may be seven months old before he does this equally well on both sides. By eight months he can locate sounds below his ear level. He does this in two stages, turning first to the appropriate side and then down to the source. Similarly by nine months he can locate sounds made above ear level in two stages. Shortly after this, location of sound becomes direct.

Interesting sounds such as footsteps, a passing car or a knock at the door instantly claim an infant's attention throughout the first year of life. After 14 or 15 months, having satisfied himself about what a particular sound means, he may subsequently ignore it.

A seven-month-old infant babbles and makes double sounds such as 'dad, dad'. At nine months he enjoys strings of babble: 'dad-dad-dad-dad!'. At 10 months he begins to practise sounds like 'bar' and 'nan', which sometimes appear to his parents to be appropriate to the situation, and may be mistakenly interpreted as the use of words with meaning. Parents' surprise and pleasure, expressed in hugs and kisses, reinforce the infant's learning.

Gross motor development

An infant of six months takes his weight on his feet with minimum support. He normally achieves a sitting posture during the next two to three weeks and

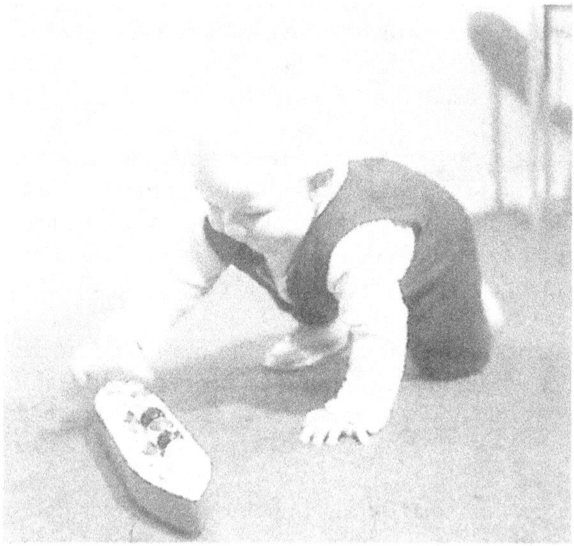

Fig. 1.5. New learning situations arise with increasing mobility.

maintains it unsupported. Saving responses become evident. Most children learn to walk from prone position. Around nine months, an infant can get into crawl posture and, stimulated by a visual attraction across the room, move towards it. A brightly coloured toy on the table or chair may catch his eye, and he is inspired to pull himself up to stand. He learns after a few bumps to control lowering himself to the ground. Next he begins to cruise around the furniture. He practises the skill to step sideways, which matures into the 'staggering' response which prevents falling when unsupported.

The moment finally comes when, with eyes ablaze with excitement and hands outstretched, the infant steps out alone. Walking is achieved first with feet far apart. Although he could get there quicker by crawling, an infant usually now chooses to walk most of the time. The urge to succeed in locomotion is, as for other pathways, a 'single step' which heralds the beginning of a new phase. The age of walking is variable and depends on family, race and culture.

Robson (1970) found that some 15 per cent of infants had a different pattern of learning to walk. In these cases there is a positive refusal even by very young babies to accept a prone posture. Sitting unsupported generally happens at a slightly later age and these infants tend to be hypotonic. They shuffle on the bottom with one or both legs flexed under; a few may roll or use a 'commando' crawl, *i.e.* pull themselves along by the arms and trail the legs. These patterns of learning to walk are usually familial.

An infant at 18 to 20 months may crawl upstairs, but soon, if his hand is held, he walks up putting both feet to each stair. He descends at first on his bottom. He climbs forwards into a nursery chair at 15 to 16 months but will soon learn to present his bottom to the seat.

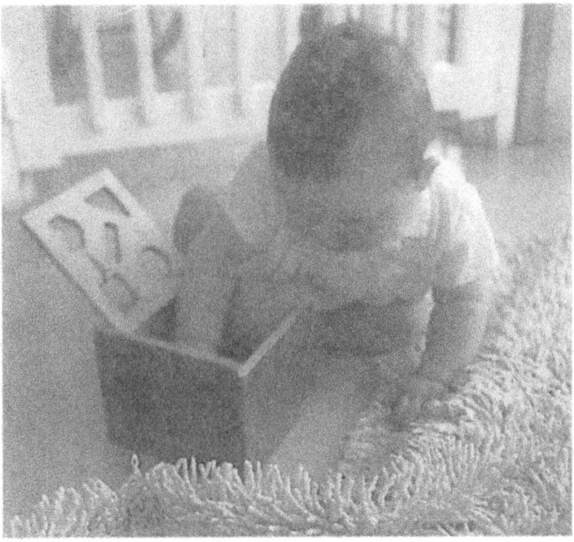

Fig. 1.6. Learning about relationships; putting in and taking out at 10 months.

Development of learning through play

A growing awareness that objects are still 'there', even when out of sight, can be demonstrated from 6½ months of age. An infant becomes aware of strangers from eight months and has to be coaxed to make a friendly relationship. By nine months he shows delight in games of 'peep-bo' across the room, moving his head in excited anticipation of mother's face reappearing from behind the curtain. If mother hides a toy under a cushion at 11 months, he finds it instantly—smiling triumphantly as he does so.

Once he is able to move at will he finds new activities for himself and his opportunities to learn are increased (Fig. 1.5). The depths of a waste-paper basket or a posting-box may be explored; he drops a toy in and retrieves it, becoming busy putting in and taking out, and thus learns the relationship of one object to another (Fig. 1.6).

Mothers commonly introduce games at nine to 12 months, helping an infant to understand gestures, situations and very simple words like 'bye-bye', 'ta' and 'pat-a-cake'. At first mother takes the child's hand to make the appropriate action, but soon a situation such as father leaving the house gives meaning to 'bye-bye'. The infant spontaneously lifts his hand, and is instantly rewarded and encouraged by his parents' show of delight.

Mother holds out her hand palm upward for a toy her infant is holding, saying 'ta' or 'give me'. He learns to respond to the gesture by offering the toy, but takes it back because he is not yet able to release from his hand. A week or so later he presses the toy down on her palm but still takes it back. By 11 months he can open his hand and leave the toy there. He has learned the skill to release through the universal habit of throwing forward, which characterises the play of the child of

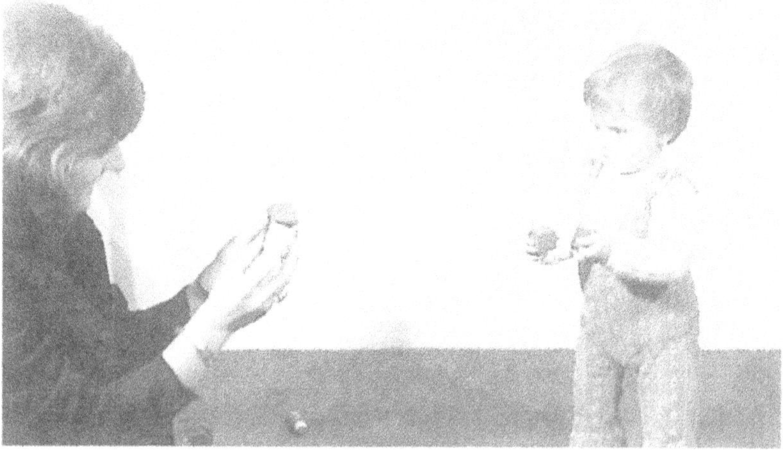

Fig. 1.7. Watching mother and learning.

nine or 10 months. During this period he learns the meaning of 'no'. On an occasion when his behaviour is unacceptable he hears 'no' and at the time sees his mother's finger raised in a warning gesture; her stance becomes a little threatening, and her face momentarily stern. He quickly learns that what he is doing is unacceptable, and the word 'no' takes on a meaning. Contrast this learning situation of an infant with normal sight with that of a severely visually-handicapped infant. He hears 'no' repeated louder and perhaps accompanied by the sound of his mother stamping her foot. The whole happening is becoming more interesting every minute, and he laughs in delight. The true meaning of 'no' is completely lost to him.

Imitation is an important factor in learning new skills. Mother clicks two bricks together. He watches carefully and soon can imitate before he learns to do it on a simple verbal demand (Fig. 1.7).

An infant at 12 months, seeing something across the room that catches his interest, flings out his arm, index finger extended, as he makes an urgent noise: 'ook' or 'der'. He is projecting himself towards the thing he desires. The pointing gesture is an important landmark in development (Fig. 1.8).

Development is expected to leap forward at the beginning of the second year in several ways. An infant spontaneously holds out his arm for his coat or his foot for his shoe. He tries to feed himself with a spoon, at first turning it upside down *en route* to his mouth. He drinks from a mug, holding it with both hands, and ducks his head as if he were diving into it. A piece of blanket may become a 'comfort' toy which must go everywhere with him. Symbolic play is beginning to emerge with everyday objects, but as yet a teddy or doll is carried as it was picked up, by its ear or foot. He will be 18 months before he carries it tenderly as he has seen his mother

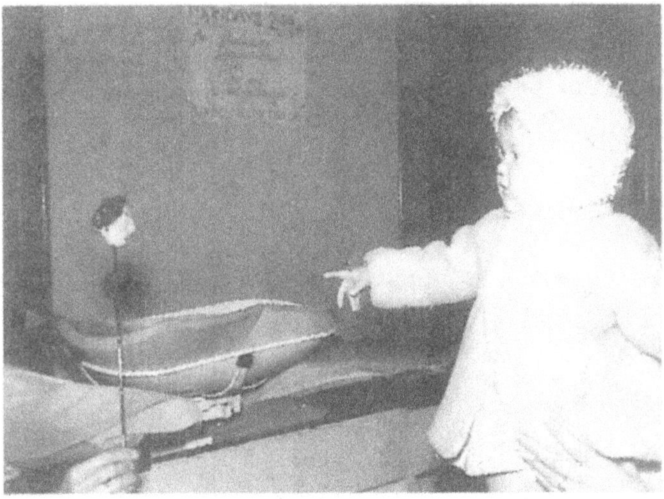

Fig. 1.8. (left). The pointing gesture.

Fig. 1.9. (below). Doll play: carrying a doll at 15 months and 20 months.

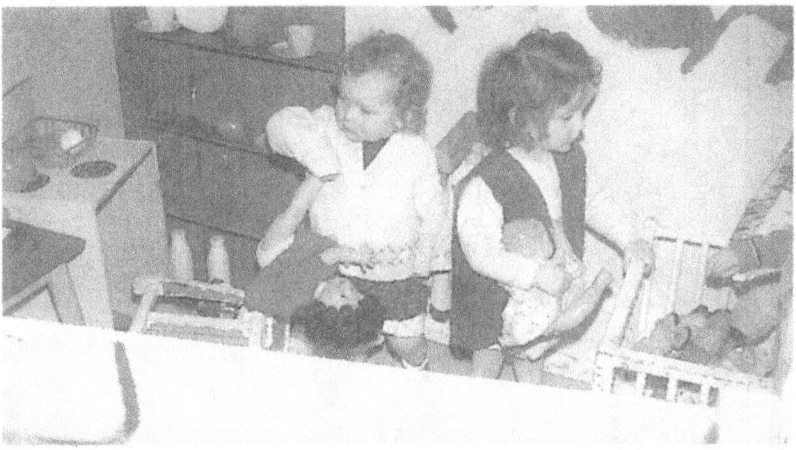

do (Fig. 1.9). He may suck at the corner of a blanket when he is tired or upset but exploration with his mouth, which was a feature in the first year, rapidly dies out.

A 14-month-old can build a tower with mother, laughing delightedly when it falls. Soon he knocks it down deliberately to enjoy the situation again—an early manifestation of a sense of humour, which is an attribute of intelligence.

The second year is a demanding time for parents as the child is utterly dependent on their almost continual attention. The child will play briefly by himself but only if mother is close at hand. Both sexes work off energy pushing a truck or pram soon filled up with an assortment of toys. Both enjoy sitting on mother's lap to look at a picture book, turning several pages together and jargoning excitedly at recognising a familiar object and soon beginning to name one or two themselves.

Parents must continually guard the active 12- to 20-month-old child from common danger which necessitates a period of high verbal input and so stimulates

TABLE 1.III

Important developmental stages: 21 months to 4½ years

				Language	
Average age	*Vision*	*Hearing*	*Performance*	*Comprehension*	*Expressive language*
21 months		Can select object from naming in quiet voice	Recognition shape Supinate pencil grasp	Symbolic play with miniature toys	Joins words to express ideas
27–33 months				Rapid advance in symbolic understanding	
33 months	Visual acuity test (adult model)			Understands questions related to experience or situations	
36 months			Tripod grasp (pencil) Draws Humpy-Dumpty Copies 3-cube bridge Copies a circle		Speech intelligible within family
39 months			Copies 4-cube train		
48 months				Begins to reason from mental image based on experience	Wholly intelligible Grammatical sentences

situational understanding: 'Don't touch that, it's hot'; 'Leave that, it will break'; 'That is Daddy's book—here is yours'; 'Don't get up there, you will fall!' A child who has a severe motor problem, or one who is severely visually handicapped and lacks the incitement to explore, may be deprived of this rich experience unless parents are advised to carry him around and teach him that some things may be touched and others may not.

The 18-month-old likes to imitate mother doing domestic chores. When she sweeps he too must have a brush. 'Helping' to wash up at the sink is an endless delight. From 20 months the child himself initiates such actions in the appropriate setting. Thus if something is spilled on the floor, he runs and fetches the dustpan and brush. He enjoys a simple inset or jigsaw puzzle, frequently demanding mother's help. Play with miniature toys (dolls' house size) becomes increasingly symbolic.

Expressive language

The way in which young children learn to express themselves in words is variable within normal limits. Some use baby words at first, *i.e.* 'brum-brum' for car. A dog may be named as 'cat' or 'horse' depending on the child's present experience. If he has a cat at home, he may, at first, name all animals as 'cat'. He is using a generic term. Piaget (1951) describes this process as assimilation, *i.e.* incorporating ideas into an existing scheme. Next he may try to express meaning by a name which conveys a function, such as 'policeman' or 'milkman'. Others omit both these stages altogether.

An advance at 20 months, which demarcates a child's level of function in expressive speech, is the ability to join words to express ideas. 'Daddy car' is an example. Substitution of consonants and difficulties with double sounds are common and may persist until three years of age when a child is expected to be wholly intelligible within his own family, although not necessarily to strangers.

Stage 3: 21 months to 4½ years (Table 1.III)

A child's understanding is dependent on his day-to-day experiences augmented by conversation, nursery rhymes, situations and simple stories. He shows understanding through gestures and in symbolic play.

From 21 months a child plays symbolically with miniature toys (dolls' house size). His play with these is at first self-related but very soon becomes detached from self, *i.e.* doll-oriented or object-to-object. These are consecutive stages in cognition but a child may, even in one short play period, revert from time to time to self-related play.

A 21-month-old is very active working off energy with pull-and-push toys, climbing or trotting about the house in almost ceaseless activity during waking hours. At two years he walks up and down stairs, holding the rail or a hand, putting both feet to each stair. At three years he alternates his feet going up. On level ground he then achieves an adult walking gait. He can imitate an adult standing on one foot.

A 21-month-old demonstrates some concept of shape and may recognise an

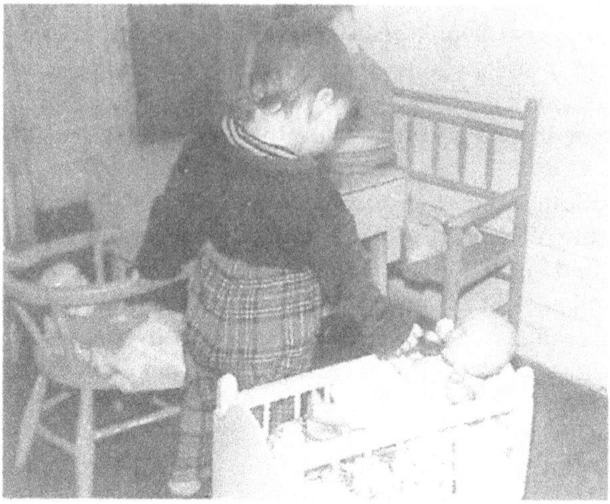

Fig. 1.10. The 'make-believe mother' at two years.

image of one or two familiar objects in the tray of an inset puzzle. A pencil is held in a supinate grasp, *i.e.* at the distal end of the pencil which is often held upright. Mother must steady the paper because a child tends to place his non-writing hand on his thigh or the table for balance. Writing will not become a two-handed operation in which the child steadies the paper for himself until after the third birthday.

A two-year-old looking at a picture selects the most significant feature, tending to fix his gaze in the middle of the visual field with only occasional excursions to the periphery. This is in marked contrast to the rapid saccadic eye movements of adults or older children (Abercrombie 1969). Once he has identified a salient feature a child then draws on his experience to show his understanding. I observed a charming example of this whilst developing the Egan bus puzzle test (see p. 56). Several high-scoring two-year-olds, when shown a post-box in a street scene, named it as 'door'. This was enigmatic until I recalled that it is a common and happy experience of young children to be lifted up to drop a letter into the box. The conspicuous feature is the slit into which he puts the letter; there is a similiar slit in his own front door. He sees it there on his eye level whenever he goes in or out. What better word could convey his understanding than 'door'?

Make-believe play occupies a child of two years for short periods. Girls tend to enjoy doll play or other domestic pursuits (Fig. 1.10). Boys, on the whole, prefer transport, and crawl about the floor pushing a car and making 'brum-brum' noises or talking to themselves. Both sexes now like to play beside their peers but not yet with them; indeed, the 30-month-old is often likely to take toys away from another child.

The attention of a two-year-old on what he is doing is fixed and rigid, and he is intolerant of help to show him how to thread a bootlace through large wooden beads. 'Me do it' is often accompanied by an impatient shrug, but soon mother is needed.

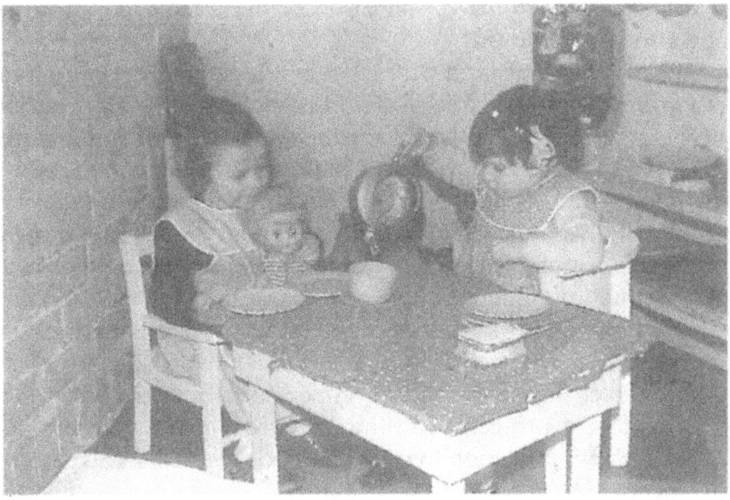

Fig. 1.11. Playing together at 2½ years.

A marked increase in symbolic understanding occurs between 27 and 33 months. Young children are helped to understand syntactical sentences about familiar situations through looking at picture books which illustrate them and from which they get situational clues. 'What is the boy doing?' becomes a question eagerly answered. Mittler (1972) described this as a kind of guesswork characteristic of normal development.

Children between 30 and 33 months show understanding of questions related to their experience. When asked 'Where do you see aeroplanes?' or when shown a picture of a boy riding a bike and asked 'What is the boy doing?' they are able to answer correctly.

The importance of parental participation in play and other activities cannot be overemphasised. A child brought up in a socially deprived home where ideas are seldom discussed is at risk of delay in language comprehension which may lead to later learning difficulties.

From 2½ years a child enjoys play for short periods with others of his own age (Fig. 1.11). At first each engages in some activity with which he is familiar, but gradually they learn from each other and extend their range. Girls may have a tea party. Two boys may make 'pies' and castles in a sandpit. They have not yet learned to share, and adult supervision must be discreetly continued. First lessons in taking turns may be learned, not without tears, in the park on swings and slides where it is necessary to wait for your turn. Painting consists of splashes of colour all over the page and crayons make great areas of scribble to be hugely enjoyed. Each 'work' has to be shown to mother or father and admired.

Three years

A three-year-old is a delightful person, happy to 'help' lay the table or to run and fetch something that has been forgotten. He is wholly intelligible in his speech to his own family but strangers may still have some difficulty. He likes to try to dress himself and soon tries to do up buttons.

He is ready for social communication with his peers. Ideally an opportunity to mix with others in a group at nursery school should be available for all preschool children whose parents wish it. It is desirable for the wide range of suitable play material including crayons, paints, scissors and plasticine, and for the outdoor equipment such as climbing frame, slide, pool and sandpit. Such amenities may be available to an only child in his own home, but there is greater value in sharing of activities with others within a group listening to stories, dressing up (usually a hat is sufficient) or acting out situations together. Kindness to others has to be learned. A three-year-old may stand and look with deep interest at another of the group who has fallen and hurt himself. A few weeks later he realises the significance of the occurrence and runs to fetch his teacher. The importance of taking turns and sharing, the development of a protective attitude towards younger or less able children, and awareness of self in relation to others, are social qualities acquired as a result of play with peers.

A three-year-old is less dependent upon immediate situations or pictures as aids to comprehension of questions within his common experience. On average, children of 36 to 39 months give a correct reply to 'Where do you see ships?' (*e.g.* 'on the water', 'in the sea' or 'on the river' (Egan and Brown 1986*b*). Contrast this with the reply of a boy over four years of age from a socially deprived home who replied 'on the telly'. He could not, despite persistent gentle probing, identify the factor which demarcates a ship from other forms of transport. At this age too a child develops concepts of time as 'now', 'tomorrow' and 'yesterday'; of quantity such as 'more' and 'lots'; and of 'sameness'. Counting is by rote and not yet related to the objects that he is supposedly counting.

A child of three years appears to be motivated to put words together as a short sentence containing a verb only when meaning cannot be imparted by a simpler form of words. Children in a highly methodical way break down language into its simplest parts and develop the rules they need to put the part together (Moskowitz 1978). When asked 'What is the lollipop man doing?' the reply 'Cross road you dead' gives you the whole dramatic story of his function in a remarkable combination of words!

Drawing

From 2½ years of age a child may try to copy the hand movements of mother drawing vertical and horizontal lines. He then holds a pencil in a *pronate* grasp—in the middle of its length with fingers flexed and thumb extended. 45 per cent of children hold a pen in this way at 30 to 33 months and then the proportion gradually declines. The *tripod* grasp—pencil held near to the point with thumb, index and middle fingers functioning together—is seen on average at 36 months. Girls are significantly better than boys in maturity of pencil grasp ($p<0.02$) (Egan and Brown 1986*a*). It is not clear whether all children necessarily go through all three stages of pencil grasp—supinate, pronate and tripod. The same child may change his grip several times in a few minutes.

TABLE 1.IV

Percentage of children with pronate or tripod grasp able to draw a cross

Age	*Pronate*	*Tripod*
42 months	38%	66%
45 months	47%	84%
48 months	75%	96%

Copying geometric shapes

Children on average can copy a circle at 36 months and a cross at 42 months. In the Egan standardisation sample, children statistically were less likely to copy a cross between the ages of 3½ and four years if their pencil grasp was immature (Table 1.IV). It is uncertain whether this reflects immaturity of both skills in demonstrating the former in the presence of the latter.

Four years

Children of four years are expected to be wholly intelligible and use gramatically correct phrases. Nouns, verbs, adjectives and pronouns are used together with other appropriate parts of speech. They are able to indicate definite preference for activities. Some may want to learn to read, others may like to have a garden plot or to look after animals. They may develop a protective attitude towards younger children and sometimes include one in their group play. Junk material or furniture is in demand to represent houses or transport, often in preference to realistic toys. They draw more and more upon reasoning based on a mental image of previous experience to comprehend questions. Past experiences are represented in group play and leadership qualities emerge especially in the context of these imaginative games. A group of some five or six children may use a crate turned upside down to become a bed, on which one becomes the patient. They clearly act out a hospital scene. They may have raided the dressing-up box to establish identities as doctor, nurses, child and parents. Dressing up is now elaborate. Their game may perhaps represent past experience. Was the leader acting out an unhappy memory? This at times can help emotional adjustment. Some caution is necessary in interpreting what children are doing—they may be merely copying a recent TV programme!

The great advantage of group experience is the enormous variety of observation and participation in diverse activities such as music, stories, climbing and gardening. Self-help, spurred on by comparison with others, the social experience of putting things away and sharing are all important. These opportunities may be available sometimes within the family or social group. But for a child living in high-rise flats, with severely limited opportunities for free play outdoors, or for the many children living in small families, the benefit of some type of play-group experience may be immeasurable.

Drawing a man

Children of three years of age attempt to draw a man. The development forms are:

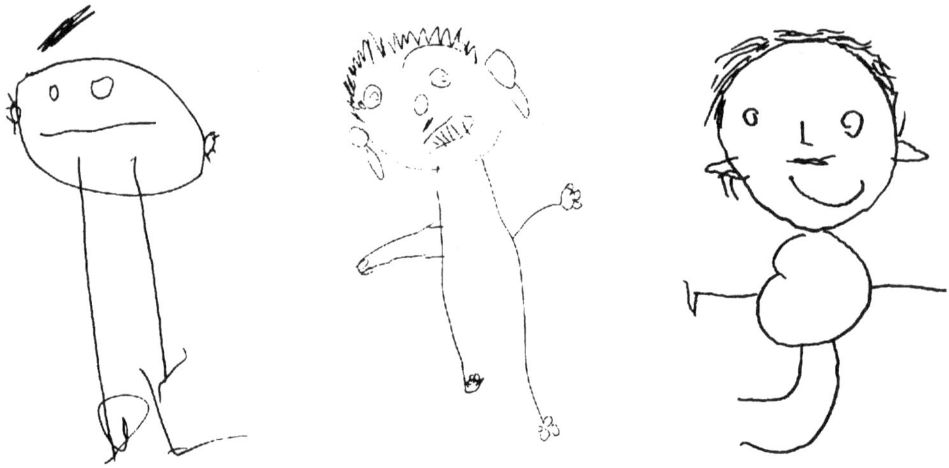

Fig. 1.12. Drawing a man. *Left:* Humpty-Dumpty. *Centre:* intermediate, and *right:* mature form.

(i) the Humpty-Dumpty man with head, no body and limbs on head, (ii) the intermediate man, again with no body but arms arising from the legs, and (iii) the mature man with head, body, and limbs on body (Fig. 1.12).

At 36 months, children on average achieve a Humpty-Dumpty man or better. The intermediate man is drawn only by a small proportion of children and it seems unlikely that all children have to go through this stage. Only 25 per cent of the author's cross-sectional sample did so. The average for drawing the mature man form was 54 months.

Copying cube models

Copying models constructed with one-inch cubes is a well known developmental sequence. Reasoning in construction is the critical skill. Children on average copy a three-cube bridge at 36 months , a four-cube train at 39 months, and six-cube steps at 4½ years (Egan and Brown 1986*a*).

2
WHEN TO WORRY ABOUT CHILDREN

'I am so worried! We live in a state of siege at home, bolts and locks on all the doors and windows! Jacky is always running away. He has been brought home by the police from stations all over Kent and Surrey. He seems mad about trains!'

I looked at the fair-haired six-year-old who sat passively beside his mother. 'He was always a lovely little lad,' she went on. 'We were buried by a land mine when he was little and were evacuated to Wales for the rest of the war. They say he is mentally deficient and will have to go to a special school.'

It was 1950. The head teacher told me that Jacky showed no interest either in lessons or in other children, and gave his teacher much trouble because he was always running away. He had been deemed mentally deficient six months previously. Regulations in force at the time required re-examination after six months if no place had been found in one of the few special schools in post-war Britain. I got out the equipment for the Terman–Merrill test. Jacky took not the slightest interest in anything I showed or said to him. After 10 minutes I was beginning to feel desperate, and I still had nothing to record. Suddenly the thought came to me, 'Trains, you fool, that is what he is interested in'. Quickly I took a sheet of drawing paper and a red pencil, and sitting on the floor began to draw a railway engine. Almost immediately he was down on the floor beside me, and snatching the pencil from my hand he began to draw! Smoke, carriages, signals and even people appeared in rapid succession. 'If this child is mentally deficient, so am I,' I thought. I knew very little of hearing tests at the time, but surely the land mine could have damaged his hearing. I arranged for him to be seen by an ear, nose and throat consultant who confirmed that Jacky was indeed severely deaf. He was admitted later to a residential school for the deaf, where as his early ability to draw had convinced me, he proved to be a highly intelligent boy.

We have advanced a long way since those post-war years when deaf children not uncommonly were sent to institutions for the mentally handicapped. The first major step was the introduction by the child health services of routine distraction tests for hearing of infants at seven or eight months of age. This expanded in the following decade into the developmental examination at key ages.

A greater interest began to be taken by hospital paediatricians in the care and management of neonates who had been born preterm, were of low birthweight, had been exposed to maternal infections such as rubella or cytomegalovirus, and who had rhesus or ABO incompatibilities or genetically determined disorders. These infants are now followed up in paediatric departments, and assessment procedures are used to determine their strengths as well as their weaknesses. Specialised techniques such as cerebral ultrasonography are now widespread throughout the country, rather than confined to a few centres of excellence as before.

The Court Report (1976) endorsed the policy of developmental 'screening' of apparently healthy children at key ages to detect as early as possible deficits which may cause learning difficulties, but visualised the work being taken over entirely by general practitioners. Their response has been uneven. The use of the term 'screening', applied to all developmental examination procedures, has perhaps led to unrealistic expectations for rapid tests which give unequivocal results. But there are complex problems to tackle: amblyopia and strabismus, intermittent hearing loss associated with middle-ear infections, language problems including those arising from social disadvantage, and reading and writing difficulties. A single developmental examination at primary-care level cannot necessarily make a full analysis of these conditions. It serves to establish that there is a developmental problem, so that a plan can be made for the guidance of parents. There may have to be further investigations by audiology or speech therapy services, paediatric or other specialist advice or some form of environmental enrichment which offers valuable observation by nursery-school teachers, psychologists and therapists, not only to arrive at a diagnosis of a child's deficits, but also to help him to reach his full potential. It is not enough to try to reassure anxious parents that 'he will grow out of it'. Child development centres for disabled children have shown the great value of team work by various disciplines. We must look for similar co-operation in the primary-care services. If it is not practical for the general practitioner to do a full development examination himself, he might arrange for the local child health services or the community paediatric team to do this for him.

Indications for developmental examination

A developmental examination is an essential part of the medical care of young children:

(1) when parents express anxiety about their young child's progress or behaviour
(2) in the management of some comparatively minor disorders of children, particularly the otitis-prone child
(3) when the doctor observes in a young child that certain patterns of behaviour expected to have been suppressed at a known age-level are persisting beyond their normal span, or
(4) when the child has a known disability.

Parental anxiety

Parents today are better informed in their expectations for their children's development, and are far more likely to consult their doctor for specific worries about their child's progress or behaviour. Parents on the whole are good observers of their children and their anxieties are often justified (Newsom 1976). It is wise to listen to what parents say.

Let us look first at the kind of worries parents bring to the doctor or health visitor, which are cues for developmental examination and the conditions that may be revealed.

Vision

The mother of a newborn baby may be anxious because he does not look at her.

This is one of the early and most dependable observations leading to suspicion that there is something wrong with an infant. Poor visual fixation and absence of visual following may be indicative of mental handicap, severe emotional problem, or even (in the absence of obvious pathology of the eyeball) of a severe vision problem. On the other hand, absence of a desire for 'bonding' with her baby may alert the doctor or midwife to postnatal depression in the mother.

A mother may report unusual movements of the baby's eyes. This is an indication for an examination of the baby's visual fixation and visual following, and observation of the baby for evidence of nystagmus. Absent or poor visual fixation and following are indicative of severe developmental problems. Nystagmus may become evident only on full dextro- or laevo-version of the eyes. Occasionally the mother may see a white patch in one eye. If examination of the eye with an ophthalmoscope at 35cm shows any impairment of the normal red reflex, immediate referral to an ophthalmologist is essential for suspected cataract, retinoblastoma or other underlying pathology.

The mother may suspect a squint. There is evidence to suggest that parents detect a squint at an earlier age than professionals, and consult their doctor, but faced by lack of medical interest some are discouraged from pursuing further ophthalmological advice. Yet a cover test can be done at any age. It is a simple procedure, but interpretation of findings needs training and practice. A persistent squint after 12 weeks of age may be indicative in the early years of underlying pathology of the eyeball. Immediate referral to an ophthalmologist is indicated.

Parents, on the other hand, rarely suspect poor visual acuity and, if strabismus and amblyopia are to be prevented, it is essential that reliable vision tests for the younger age-groups are developed.

Hearing

Three categories of hearing problems are discussed:
(1) congenital hearing loss
(2) hearing loss associated with infectious diseases, and
(3) hearing loss associated with middle-ear infections.

1. CONGENITAL HEARING LOSS

A mother may notice that her baby does not seem to be aware of her approach to his cot, and looks startled when her face appears. She may complain that he seems unaware of normal sounds (the doorbell ringing or a low-flying aeroplane) and yet notices immediately when someone comes into the room. The congenitally deaf baby is often very visually alert. Congenital hearing loss is a severe handicap because the infant does not hear speech. There have been considerable advances recently in earlier diagnosis, due to more positive reactions by primary-care doctors to mothers' anxieties about children's hearing (Davies 1988). The use of an auditory response cradle in some neonatal departments has led to diagnosis of congenital hearing loss in the first days of life. Immediate treatment is now often possible because of enormous technological advances in the design and quality of hearing-aids for very young infants.

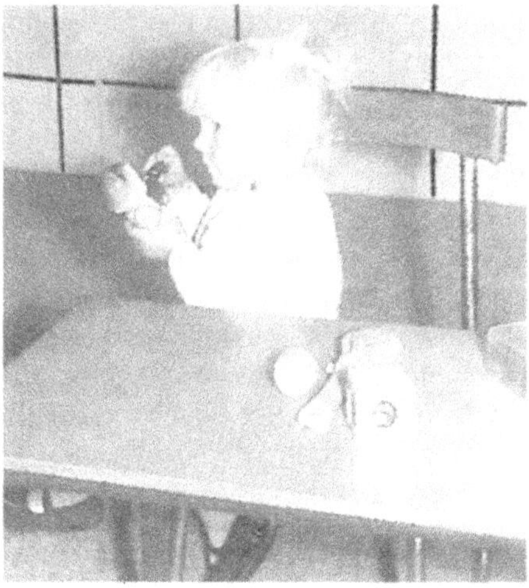

Fig. 2.1. A profoundly deaf child shows symbolic play at two years.

When congenital hearing loss is suspected, a full developmental examination is important because the future management of the child may depend on his potential in other areas. A case history may serve to illustrate this point.

A two-year-old girl had been brought to the hospital clinic because she had no speech. A full developmental assessment was about to begin, and the child was seated at a nursery table. The staff had earlier been taking photographs, and while she waited, she saw a discarded flash-bulb lying on the table. The little girl picked up the bulb and began to feed her doll with it (Fig. 2.1). This spontaneous make-believe situation, in which the tiny glass bulb represented to her a baby's feeding bottle, demonstrated vividly that the child's comprehension was at the expected level for her age. Ability to symbolise with miniature toys normally emerges at 20 to 22 months of age. This little girl clearly had good potential. Investigation revealed a profound congenital hearing loss.

2. HEARING LOSS ASSOCIATED WITH INFECTIOUS DISEASES

Hearing loss may be associatd with infectious diseases of childhood, such as measles, mumps or meningitis. This complication is not common, but should be borne in mind when changes in behaviour arouse parental anxiety. A little girl three years of age seemed unwell. She was off her food and was lying on the sofa cuddling her doll. Coincidentally the health visitor called that day to see the six-week-old baby brother. She was asked to see the little girl but was not unduly worried as there was only a mild rise of temperature. The next day the child appeared to her mother to have completely recovered. But as the weeks went by the mother became increasingly worried because this previously happy busy little girl became more and more wilful, continually banging doors or scraping the kitchen chairs along the stone floor of the kitchen; refusing to answer questions and given to outbursts of temper. Was she jealous of the new baby? Eventually the mother consulted her doctor. Clinical tests of hearing revealed a profound hearing loss which had followed a mild illness, possibly viral meningitis. The child was referred to the audiology centre. It was essential to try to preserve her comprehension of language. A radio-link hearing-aid was prescribed for use in her home and in her nursery school.

3. THE OTITIS-PRONE CHILD

Middle-ear effusions are a common disorder of childhood even in the very young. Infection in the nose and throat may readily spread to the middle ear. Enlarged adenoids are often present.

The child initially complains of pain in the ear which may respond to treatment with antibiotics. Parents unfortunately are not always reliable in completing a full course of medicinal treatment, or become less so if their child is constantly catarrhal. Antihistamines may be given over a period of time as an alternative treatment, especially for children with an allergic history. The long-term results of either treatment are variable and chronic serous otitis media may sometimes develop, giving rise to a hearing loss which tends to be worse in the lower frequencies. The hearing loss may be temporary, or may be longer term. 17 per cent of children have a hearing loss some time after an attack of otitis media (Fry 1970).

Parents do not appear to suspect deafness in children with conductive hearing loss. A mother's response when questioned about the child's hearing is typical: 'He can hear all right if he wants to!' This exactly describes the child's problem—a difficulty to pay sustained attention until mother in exasperation raises her voice above 50db. It might usefully be regarded by doctors as a signal to do a clinical test of hearing. Children under two years of age who have 'glue' ears are at high risk of language delay. Children over three are likely to have learning difficulties and emotional problems. Hamilton and Owrid (1974), reporting on the effects of hearing impairment on verbal attainments, showed that hearing loss including conductive deafness was a more serious handicap for linguistic skills such as reading than socio-cultural factors. Thus educational disadvantages are decided before the child reaches school.

A young child with variable hearing loss is at risk not only of learning difficulties but, if the condition is undiagnosed at school age, of loss of self-confidence and behavioural difficulties.

Let us follow David, who has unsuspected chronic serous otitis media, into his primary school. There is no longer a focal point for teaching in the classroom. The teacher goes round the tables, at each of which some four to six children are sitting, to give individual reading lessons. Today it is David's turn. The teacher stands behind him and her voice comes to David from behind his head, a situation from which it is most difficult to hear. Ambient noise from classmates busy with other tasks increases his difficulty. The effort to sustain attention becomes too great. As the weeks go by David realises that his peers are beginning to read and he is not. Confidence in himself is a little shaken. At home he soon begins to sense his parents' disappointment. 'I wonder why David is slow in learning to read? Diana was reading quite well in her second term and she was in Miss Blank's class!' A consultation may be arranged with the head teacher and, as sometimes may happen, David's mother may be mystified to hear that he has not got 'reading readiness'. 'Why hasn't he?' demands his exasperated father.

The keen observer of child behaviour will be aware that a prolonged sense of failure can have an adverse effect on a young child's will to master his environment, and in the long term may induce a lack of self-confidence as well as associated behaviour problems. These effects can persist long after the original infection has cleared up. Partial deafness from otitis media and glue ear was reported in 31 per 1000 children from birth to four years (Rutter *et al.* 1970).

There is controversy whether the results of surgical treatment (grommets) are better than the more conservative treatment with antibiotics and/or antihistamines (Brown *et al.* 1978). Parents may cease antibiotic therapy as soon as the acute symptoms disappear; antihistamine therapy is often very long-term and may be effective only when the infection has an allergic origin; the affected child may often require adenoidectomy. If general practitioners could be persuaded as a routine to recall the child at (say) eight weeks after therapy for ear infections, to make a clinical test of hearing, and refer those who have a hearing loss to the audiology centre for an impedance test or follow-up, this might be a valuable first step towards identifying children whom we should worry about. Teachers could be informed so that the child is placed in favourable conditions for learning.

Language

Parents may be worried if the infant is late in beginning to talk, if speech is not intelligible (sometimes leading to tantrums), or occasionally because their child is beginning to stammer. Thus parents observe delay or something unusual in *expressive* speech, and this is what they describe to the doctor. But language is not simply speech. Language is communication. The cognitive factor is comprehension. Comprehension and expressive speech must be looked at separately. A profile of language and performance skills can reveal a development problem.

The common causes of language delay are:

(1) mental handicap
(2) deafness
(3) severe social deprivation, and
(4) specific language disorders.

Other less common causes are severe vision problems; infantile autism, which is rare; and structural problems of lips, tongue or palate, or motor disorders involving these. Stammering in its true sense is rare in the under-fives. The hesitations and repetitions of the two- to three-year-old are likely to be part of the developmental process in joining words to express ideas. Parents should be advised to ignore them, or at most to help out with a word.

1. MENTAL HANDICAP

This may be of varying degree. If achievement is substantially below average (lowest 10th centile) across the language/performance profile, this is suggestive of mental handicap—mild to more severe.

2. DEAFNESS
A careful assessment of hearing is essential in *every* case of suspected language delay. Congenital hearing loss causes profound language delay. Middle-ear infections in infants under two years of age may lead to substantial delay; learning difficulties and emotional problems are more common in the over-threes.

3. SEVERE SOCIAL DEPRIVATION
Children living in severely socially deprived homes may be identified by their general practitioner as those brought repeatedly to him for upper respiratory infections, recurrent gastro-enteritis, or recurring accidents in the home or street. A developmental examination may reveal a poor grasp of language right across the language base, but not to wide discrepancies within the profile. Bax *et al.* (1990) found that 20 per cent of children attending their health clinic suffered respiratory problems, developmental delay and behavioural problems, closely associated with adverse social findings. Some form of environmental enrichment, a nursery school or play-group, needs to be augmented by a follow-up by the health visitor in the home to teach the mother ways in which she can help; or by speech therapy, together with a programme for mother to carry out on a daily basis.

4. SPECIFIC DEVELOPMENTAL LANGUAGE DISORDERS
There are two groups of specific language disorders, *i.e.* a primary constitutional disorder, and secondary to brain damage. Family history is important in the former group. Sonksen (1979) found that the occurrence rate in males was high (1 in 3.7). Genetic advice may be helpful to such families. The language behaviour of younger siblings should be carefully monitored by a speech therapist.

Performance skills
Parents may complain that their child is clumsy: 'I never let him help lay the table, he always drops things', 'He is no good at ball games', or 'He cannot do up buttons'.

Clumsiness has been defined as 'a deficit in the acquisition of skills requiring fluent or ordered movement, not explicable by general retardation or demonstrable neurological disease' (Hall 1988).

When clumsiness is evident to parents they express considerable anxiety about the child's future progress. There may be a family history of late reading, poor spelling and/or writing skills, especially in male members of the family. Is this child going to have similar difficulties when he goes to school? Are these patterns of behaviour predictive of later specific reading and writing problems? Francis-Williams (1976), in a follow-up study of early identification of children likely to have specific learning difficulties, found that over-all poor or delayed language development is an indication of later learning difficulties at school. We cannot draw any positive conclusions without more long-term studies, but we can at least recognise the pattern of behaviour as deviant development, and a pointer for developmental examination. There is some evidence that these children do benefit from admission to a nursery school and the expert help of a skilled nursery-school teacher.

Gross motor skills

Parents may be worried because their child is 'late' in walking. The age of walking is very variable, and unless there is evidence of either a motor disorder or dislocation of the hip, there is probably little cause for worry before 18 months of age. There are two categories of late walkers (Chaplais and Macfarlane 1984): idiopathic and symptomatic.

Idiopathic late walkers have a different pattern of learning to walk (see p. 8). The diagnosis depends on: (i) a normal obstetric history, (ii) strong family history of shuffling, and (iii) moderate hypotonia. A characteristic sitting posture on the floor is common, *i.e.* between the knees with feet at hip level; marked joint mobility with hyperextension of knee joints and plano-valgus feet. When the downward parachute reaction is elicited at seven or eight months, the child assumes a sitting posture. One variant in some 'shuffling' families is that the first-born child may at about 10 months of age simply stand up and walk.

Symptomatic late walking may be due to dislocation or subluxation of hip, or diplegia or other neuromotor disorder. Diagnosis may be helped by:

(1) a history of difficult labour or adverse perinatal conditions, no family history of shuffling, and assessment of motor function to reveal signs of neuromotor disorder, and
(2) Ortolani-Barlow test in infants up to four months of age; examination of hip joint.

It must be remembered that occasionally a child in a shuffling family may also have a motor disorder. The diagnosis is then more difficult and may require expert opinion. Mental handicap may be a cause of late walking because walking is a learned process. A full developmental examination will reveal substantial delay in the language/performance profile.

Patterns of behaviour persisting beyond their normal span

Certain patterns of behaviour of young infants emerge at a known age-level, persist for a period and are then suppressed. Persistence of these patterns of behaviour beyond their normal span is significant and suggests that there may be a developmental problem.

These behaviours are useful indicators for developmental examination, if present after specific ages have been reached:

(1) hand regard
(2) exploration of all toys in the mouth, and
(3) casting behaviour.

Hand regard is a normal pattern of behaviour which emerges from 12 weeks of age when a baby first begins to control his visual attention on his fingers held close to his face. This reaches a peak between 16 and 20 weeks then virtually disappears as a substantial activity from six months.

Persistence of hand regard from eight months of age suggests a developmental problem which may be some degree of mental handicap or a severe visual problem. Allowance should be made in preterm infants for the period of gestation.

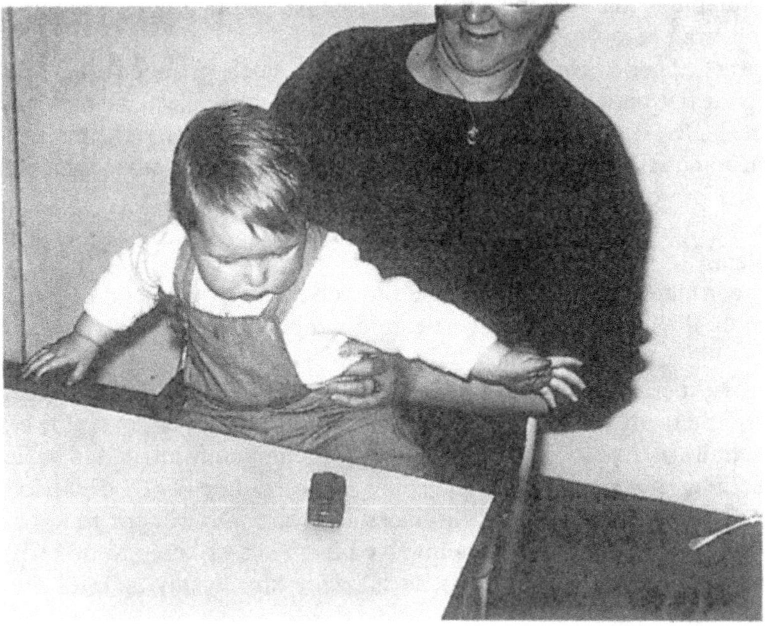

Fig. 2.2. Casting; normal behaviour at 13 months.

Exploration of toys in the mouth. An infant in the first year, from birth to 13 months of age, normally explores in his mouth any object put into his hand or picked up. This behaviour sharply declines from 13 months of age.

A child who is tired or distressed may *at any age* suck his thumb, the corner of his 'comfort' blanket or a toy. This is a normal momentary reversion to more immature behaviour under stress. The experienced doctor in these circumstances will know how to set up a more relaxed relationship with the child. If *all* toys on presentation are immediately taken to the mouth rather than used in meaningful play, at 18 months of age, the question must arise of serious delay in a child's level of understanding.

Casting behaviour (Fig. 2.2). An infant in the second year of life uses to the full his new-found mobility to explore his environment. He takes down anything within reach, looks intently at it, feels it and turns it about, until his interest fades, when he casts it behind him without a backward glance and goes on to other interests.

This is normal behaviour characteristic of the period from 12 to 18 months, after which it rapidly disappears. Persistence of casting behaviour from 20 months onwards is significant and may indicate a learning disability.

The child with a known disability

Multiple disabilities are more common than single ones. A child who has a congenital developmental disability or impairment is at high risk of other hidden problems. An example is the high incidence of refractive errors of vision found in children suffering from cerebral palsy.

A general practitioner or child health doctor cannot safely assume that a child who is attending an out-patient hospital department for (say) a right hemiplegia, has necessarily had a full development examination there. All too often he has not.

A child with a known congenital handicap is in need of periodic developmental examination in the preschool years.

Behaviour problems

Doctors may be consulted by parents because the behaviour of the child becomes disruptive to family life. The common worries are sleeping, temper tantrums and food fads.

Some parents experience difficulty in getting a young baby to settle to sleep when put down. Others are troubled because a child wakes once or several times every night, especially in the second year of life. This is commonly attributed to the discomfort of teething, but can be very disturbing and cannot be lightly dismissed. Other families may experience extreme wilfulness in a child who will not go to bed without his parents. Some get themselves involved in rituals of going to bed with the child and getting up when he is asleep, or allowing him to stay up until they themselves go to bed.

The child in the second year of life becomes increasingly aware of his power to control situations. This is normal developmental progress, but at times can become very threatening to the peace of the family. Food fads may be carried to bizarre lengths, so that meal-times which should be a social event become instead a battle ground. Very real anxiety may arise when this is carried to extreme lengths so that the child becomes at risk of under-nourishment. Others may develop temper tantrums, and scream and fuss several times a day, and so embarrass their parents that, in desperation, they give in to the child's demands. The incidence of severe behavioural problems is high. Jenkins *et al.* (1984), in a study of behavioural problems in preschool children, found that 16 per cent of three-year-olds had poor appetite and 12 per cent were described as very faddy. Temper tantrums were found in 5 to 9 per cent of two-year-olds, 18 per cent of three-year-olds, and remained as high as 11 per cent in children at 4½ years of age. Correlations were found between language and speech delay and behavioural problems (Stevenson and Richman 1976).

Time-honoured measures may well be inappropriate when behaviour problems threaten the integrity of the family. A long and careful history, supplemented by observation in the home itself, can be carried out by an experienced health visitor. It is important to establish whether both parents are equally anxious to bring about change, or whether one is more tolerant, or perhaps fearful of the effects of appropriate alterations in management because these might upset the child. Some situations may require investigation and the advice of a psychologist as well as the deployment of other local agencies.

3
THE CRAFT OF DEVELOPMENTAL EXAMINATIONS

Over the many years of evolving skills and tests needed for developmental examinations I watched the behaviour of young children when brought by worried parents. The baby was either asleep, or mother was occupied in giving him a bottle to ensure that he dropped off. A young child just fidgeted with boredom while grown-ups talked, then showed immediate alarm when later he was addressed by a stranger. The aim is to try to ensure that the baby is awake and the child contentedly occupied during the history-taking.

It is useful perhaps to begin by giving some thought to the arrangement of the consulting room as far as its constraints will allow. If the doctor is seated behind a desk, its paraphernalia—papers, pens, books and instruments—can be powerful visual distractions to the very young; or because it distances him from the child, can create a barrier to the play situation he seeks to contrive.

The following items of furniture are suggested:

1. A small square table of suitable height that an infant of six months sitting supported on mother's lap can look down at small toys placed on it. It is an added advantage if the surface is covered with adhesive matt black material against which coloured toys have a maximum visual attractiveness.

2. A nursery table with a similar covered surface; a nursery chair, preferably with arms, which gives a sense of security and serves to keep a small child penned in, when a momentary loss of concentration or shyness excites a sudden desire for mother's lap. An inspired physiotherapist colleague attached a step to the chair used for many years. It was a continual delight to generations of small children who climbed into it!

3. A small chest of drawers is useful for placing out of sight toys which have already been used while the next procedure takes place.

4. A small mattress for very young babies, and a foam mat for the examination of gross motor development of infants.

Making a social relationship with a child

When greeting parents, do not forget to include even the smallest baby. The six-month-old is friendly and outgoing and readily responds to a kindly approach. The infant of eight months is becoming aware of strangers, hence advances have to be gradual and may take a little longer. The task may seem a little daunting if one is faced with a not-very-willing youngster, but there are strategies which make this easier. Avoid 'What is your name?' or 'How old are you, my boy?' which often prove disastrous. Know the child's name and use it. As you drop down to his level a quick glance will reveal a useful feature to divert attention—'What a pretty dress! I see it's got pockets (buttons, collar)'. This is a prelude to 'Would you like to come with Mummy to see my toys?'

The child during history-taking

A relationship already begun should not be allowed to evaporate while the history is being taken. A little foresight may help to ensure that the child remains occupied until his examination begins.

A six-week-old baby must be observed when awake. There is no way you can assess a sleeping baby. Cocooned in a shawl against his mother's chest he will certainly be in a deep sleep. As a first step, suggest that mother removes his outer clothing. Place him on a small mattress and perhaps put a toy in his hand. A brightly coloured rattle is useful for the infant of over three months. Does he hold it? Pass it from one hand to the other? Does he visually track it as it falls to the floor? Does the 10-month-old visually search for it? You can observe these actions as you talk to mother.

The child from 13 or 14 months should be encouraged to sit in the nursery chair rather than on mother's lap. Catch his attention with a wooden boat with detachable peg-men. Observe his play when he is left to himself. Does he jargon as he pushes the boat to and fro? Does he take the peg-men out and replace them competently, or does he simply put one in his mouth?

Wooden jigsaw puzzles* will prove invaluable for children of two years upwards. Note the strategies the child uses to solve the puzzle. Is he absorbed in trying to fit the pieces together? Does he constantly demand mother's attention? How does she cope with the situation while trying to give her mind to the history-taking? This brief insight into family attitudes and relationships is sometimes in itself of value. It is also a subtle way to begin a relationship with a child.

Toys which are actual test material should *never* be given to the child in this preliminary play situation.

Management of the child in a developmental examination

Once the developmental examination itself begins, talk to the child in simple language as their parents do, and as you would speak to your own child of the same age. Raise your voice slightly to command attention. Use simple words and grammar which a child of this age can be expected to understand. 'What is it?' is what mother says to a two-year-old, *not* 'What is it called?' Avoid that awkward pause that allows a child to become suddenly aware of his strange surroundings and retreat into mother's shoulder or get down from his chair. A relationship once lost often proves difficult to restore.

If a child gives a wrong answer, never say 'no'. Either repeat your question or change the subject with an encouraging remark 'What a clever boy (girl) you are! Shall we look at something else? I will show you my best toy!' Young children are sensitive to failure just as much as they are pleased with success.

*These puzzles of graded difficulty can be obtained from Galt Toys, 84 Fortis Green Road, London N10 3HN, and Hurst's Toys, Unit 8, North Street Workshops, Stoke-sub-Hamdon, Somerset TA14 6QR.

Attention control

There is a developmental sequence according to age in a child's ability to stop what he is doing, to listen to what you say and then to carry out your instruction (Cooper *et al.* 1978).

Doctors need to know how to control an infant's attention, to direct it gently to another situation without causing a crisis; and when to expect a child to do this on a verbal direction.

A marked delay in the expected level of attention control at any age may of itself be a pointer to a developmental problem.

Sequence of attention control

BIRTH TO 13 MONTHS

Attention control is brief up to 13 months of age. An infant is immediately distracted by any external stimulus such as a voice, movement, or noise of a passing car or aeroplane. A reasonably quiet room is clearly desirable but sound-proofing is not necessary at primary-care level. It is useful to observe the way in which the young infant reacts to stimuli in an everyday situation.

14 TO 19 MONTHS

Remember that the infant's attention on an object of choice is fixed and not easily diverted. He will not willingly give up a toy which has aroused his interest. The 14- or 15-month-old, for example, can select a toy named to him from a choice of three or four on the table. It has then to be taken gently from his hand before he can choose another named to him. If he is allowed to hold the toy he will have attention only for it and ignore you. I banished toy cars entirely from my equipment—the attention of little boys on a miniature car is utterly inflexible!

20 TO 30 MONTHS

The child of 20 months enters a transient stage of attention control. A natural eagerness to explore a new situation must be controlled because it can only be channelled on one thing at a time. He can briefly transfer attention away from what he is doing only if his visual and auditory attention are demanded and held. Place your hands lightly over his to encourage him to listen. Look him in the eye, and speak slowly and simply before releasing his hands to carry out your instruction. You must completely control the situation and re-set the child's attention for each new instruction.

31 TO 47 MONTHS

The child still concentrates on one thing but is beginning to learn to control his attention. He can sometimes pause and listen to a verbal instruction before refocusing attention on carrying it out. This ability increases with age. He may however revert to a more immature pattern, from time to time. If he does so, gently restrain his hands and so recapture his attention.

48 MONTHS

The four-year-old can from time to time take in an instruction without stopping what he is doing and incorporate the direction given to him.

The parents

You will wish one or both of the parents to be present while the developmental examination is carried out. If both are present try to sit both on the *same* side of the child. This effectively prevents a child 'playing off' one parent against the other—a not uncommon characteristic of little girls!

The presence of parents is in itself an advantage because it enables them to see for themselves what the child is able to do. They may be surprised by some new skill: 'I didn't know Sam/Jane could do that'. Others may be disappointed that some skills are less than their expectations. Either situation offers an opportunity for advice about books, play material to help develop skills, or encouragement to allow more contact with his peers.

The aim, while holding the child's attention on the task in hand, is to allow the child to feel secure that the mother is there, although not at the level of his immediate consciousness. She must be firmly discouraged from offering her help or exhorting the child to try harder. It may sometimes be necessary to ask in passing: 'Do you say "clap hands" or "pat-a-cake"?' or when you sense in her a rising anxiety about the basic question: 'I don't expect him to do this'.

Sometimes a child, commonly in the second year of life, may refuse to sit in the chair and resist all encouragement to begin to play even a simple game of building cubes. Do not take what appears to be the easy option, to let the child sit on mother's lap. Let him stand. If he still resists persuasion to build, bring mother into the situation temporarily as an ally: 'Mummy will help me. Would you like to put a brick on the top, Mummy?' The child must then be completely ignored by both of you for the next minute or two, while you build in turn and talk. Suddenly you hold out your hand to him, 'Give me a brick. I'll put it on for you.' If he responds, a relationship with you has begun and soon he will be building too.

A crucial moment for anxious parents comes when the examination is finished and they look for the doctor's opinion. Remember that the intention is not to predict future intelligence or success but to determine whether the child is developing normally for his age (Illingworth 1970). If the child's achievements are average or above it is encouraging to select something that he does well: 'He is very good at building models' or 'He expresses himself very clearly'. It is wise to resist the temptation to be predictive! On the other hand if a developmental problem is suspected, parents may have to be persuaded of the necessity for further advice or treatment, or you yourself may wish to make a follow-up appointment. Sometimes parents may be a little illogical, for example a mother may be dismayed that her pretty daughter may have to wear glasses and unwilling for this reason to seek the advice of an ophthalmologist or optician.

Again, for a child whose achievements are below average, parents must from the beginning be helped to realise that some form of therapy or environmental enrichment, such as a nursery school or play-group, may be helpful but will need their back-up. This must include the way they talk at home about how and why they do things when out shopping or in the park.

4
A PLAN FOR DEVELOPMENTAL EXAMINATION

The plan for a developmental examination divides into three age-groups: (i) birth to six months, (ii) seven to 20 months, and (iii) 21 months to 4½ years.

A basic plan includes:

(1) history

(2) clinical tests of hearing

(3) visual behaviour or visual acuity

(4) gross motor behaviour

(5) a language/performance profile. In the first six months this aspect is directed mainly to making sure that social communication between mother and baby is being established. Thereafter any substantial unevenness, or over-all low scores in the profile, may reveal a developmental problem

(6) a physical examination to include head circumference, length/height and weight measurements, as well as tests for dislocation of hips, a check for undescended testes, and auscultation of heart and lungs. (The reader is referred to textbooks of general paediatrics for details of physical examination. A standard head-circumference chart with which to compare the pattern of head growth of the individual child is essential. In our multi-racial society some variation from standard measurements is to be expected, but the over-all growth pattern should follow the standard.)

Allowance for preterm birth should always be made in the first year. In the second year, delay in the language/performance profile requires further observation from 16 or 17 months of age.

Clinical tests of hearing should always be carefully repeated in every instance of language delay.

History

This includes a full history of pregnancy, labour and the puerperium, family structure and birth rank of child. Are the parents first cousins, and is there any known handicap?

Hearing

What do parents think of the child's hearing? Are there any middle-ear infections in the child, and is there a history of hearing loss?

Vision

What is the parental view of the child's vision? Did the baby look at mother when feeding? Does he watch animals or birds? Where does the child sit to watch TV? Is there a family history of squint, wearing glasses or other eye problems?

TABLE 4.I

Developmental examination: six weeks to 27 weeks

History			
Hearing test			*Response*
6 weeks	Gently shake small bell 15cm from ear on ear level		Stilling and eye widening
16 weeks	Stroke back of spoon on rim of cup at 90cm from ear on ear level		Head turning but *not* visual location of sound source
Vision			
6 weeks	Pupil reaction; red reflex; visual fixation and visual following		
12 weeks	Persistent squint is significant		
Gross motor			
6 weeks	Pulled to sit—head support 3 sec: ventral suspension—head in line with back; elbows flexed; some hip extension Ortolani-Barlow test for dislocation of hips Primitive responses present pass off at four months		
20 weeks	Held upright and tipped off balance spontaneous balancing reactions		
22 weeks	Legs up in vertical		
24 weeks	Picks up cube Palmar grasp Takes weight on feet with minimum support		
Social communication			*Performance*
6 weeks	Social smile	Soft vocalisations	
12 weeks	Finger play close to face	Vowel sounds	
16 weeks	Hand regard		Reaches for suspended toy
18 weeks	Visual attention on flexed knees		
20 weeks		Responsive vocalisations	
22 weeks	Visual attention on feet in vertical	Loud sounds; blows raspberries	Grasps foot to put in mouth Pats with flat hand in unco-ordinated attempt to pick up toy on table

Motor
At what age were developmental milestones achieved (sitting, standing and walking) and are there any unusual or clumsy movements?

Language/performance
How much does the child understand? How does he let you know what he wants: by vocalising or using expressive speech? And is there any family history of speech problems?

Does he achieve what parents expect for age? Can he amuse himself? Is there any history of reading or writing difficulties in the family?

The examiner should also take into account the child's emotional state and behaviour problems; his environment; the health visitor's report of the home and parenting skills; and how the parents describe their child.

Guidance for action
Developmental examination procedures are carried out in a contrived play situation in which a child is encouraged to give of his best. A broad knowledge of normal development and of age-levels when certain skills are expected to appear is essential for the interpretation of findings.

Time factor
It is now widely recognised that skills in developmental examination require training and repeated practice. The time factor is commonly underestimated. This may lead to unacceptable short cuts. A realistic appraisal of the time likely to be required, related to the age of the child, is overdue. A developmental examination of an infant under 12 months of age may be completed by an experienced examiner in 10 to 15 minutes. A child of 13 months upwards has to be persuaded to give active co-operation and to maintain it throughout the examination. It is seldom possible to complete this task in less than 20 minutes. A further five to 10 minutes should be allowed for history-taking; a physical examination and for discussion with parents of the health education aspects which often arise, even in the management of children who appear to be developing normally. When developmental delay is revealed, parents have not only to be informed of the deficit but also guided about services available to help the child, as well as their vital role in any remedial treatment. Some parents may be deeply anxious, asking 'Will he go to school?'—in other words, to 'normal' school. It is a poignant reminder that sometimes parental fears are profound.

Developmental examination procedures for hearing and hearing behaviour, vision, gross motor skills, and for establishing a profile of language and performance skills, are described in detail in later chapters.

Six weeks to six months
The establishment of social communication with mother; examination of visual behaviour; response to sound, and the development of gross motor skills are examined. Any substantial delay is significant (allowing for preterm birth)—*e.g.* absence of the smiling response at eight or nine weeks (Table 4.I).

TABLE 4.II

Developmental examination: seven months to 19 months

History

Hearing Distraction tests, 1m on ear level. Voiced sounds 'ss-ss' 'oo-oo'. Low speech—turns to locate source of sound

Visual behaviour Ball on string. Visual fixation and following. Look for full abduction. Cover test for strabismus

	Profile			
	Language		*Performance*	
	Comprehension	*Expressive language*	*Fine manipulation*	*Visuo-perceptual skills*
			Two cubes on table	
				*Roll ball and flip over table edge**
				Holds gaze at point of going
7 months		'Dad-dad'	Picks up two. Explores with index finger	Moves to look for ball (1 : 3 times)
9 months		Babbles in strings	Explores with index finger 3 : 3	Moves to look for ball (3 : 3 times)
	'Give me'		*'Give me'*	
10 months	Offers		Offers, takes back	
10½ months		Imitative babble	Presses on palm, takes back	
11 months			Finger release	
	Familiar objects larger than miniature			
13 months	Definition by use			Cubes—begins to build
14–15 months	Hands correctly on request	Jargons		
15–20 months		Naming 5/6		

*Some doubt has been raised whether there is a cognitive element.

Gross motor skills

Age for sitting and crawling is variable. Downward parachute-sitting posture suggests shuffling syndrome

15 months	Squats and rises to standing without support
18 months	Walking unless family history of shuffling
	Examine hips for subluxation if walking is delayed

TABLE 4.III

Developmental examination: 20 months to 4½ years

History		
Hearing	Doll features and large toys McCormick's toy discrimination test Stycar picture tests (6 and 12)	named in a low voice
Visual behaviour	Abduction of eyes—ball on string test Cover test for strabismus Sonksen picture test from 20 months	
Visual acuity	Sonksen/Silver acuity system with occlusion—from 3½ years Egan/Calver linear chart and plastic letters with occlusion—from 3½ years	
Gross motor	Rise to standing from squat from 15 months. Throws and kicks ball from two years; stands on one foot at three years	

Profile

Language			*Performance*	
Comprehension	*Expressive language*		*Fine manipulation*	*Visuo-perceptual skills*
		Egan bus puzzle test		
Verbal labels (9)		30 months		Recognition of shape (9)
Qs on situations (6)	Verbal labels (9)	36 months		Orientation of pieces (9)
	Answers to questions (sentences)	48 months		
		Cube models test		
		33–36 months		Copies bridge
		39 months		Copies train
		54 months		Copies 3-cube steps
		33–36 months	Pencil grasp—tripod	Copies circle
		39–42 months		Copies cross
		51 months		Copies square
		Draw-a-man test		
		36 months		Humpty-Dumpty man
		54 months		Mature man

Guidance for action: figures given in the profile show when 50 per cent of children achieve the skill.
There is an average range of achievement, lowest 20 per cent identified as children requiring further follow-up or investigation.

Seven months to 19 months

The essentials of a developmental examination are clinical tests of hearing: examination of a visual behaviour and of developing gross motor skills; development of comprehension and of expressive language, and the acquisition of fine manipulation and visuo-motor skills. Any substantial variation in expected responses (*i.e.* four weeks, allowing for preterm birth) requires further follow-up or investigation (Table 4.II).

20 months to 4½ years

Children in this age range can co-operate in more sophisticated clinical tests for hearing; and from 33 months in tests of visual acuity. Any substantial unevenness or an over-all low score in the language performance profile may reveal a developmental problem. Comprehension and expressive language are scored separately, and performance skills recorded as fine manipulation and visuo-perceptive skills.

It is necessary to define what is meant by 'substantial unevenness' and what should be regarded as an over-all low score. There is a wide range of normal ability. The 50th centile for any particular skill is not, of itself helpful in coming to a decision whether or not action should be taken. It is necessary to define a level of achievement below which developmental delay is significant.

Normal distribution curves provide a 10-point scale in which persons whose skills are in the 4 to 7 point range are defined as 'average'. Those whose skills fall below 4 (*i.e.* the lowest 16 per cent) are definitely below average (Cattell 1982).

We can extrapolate from this specialised field that children whose skills in the language/performance profile fall into the lowest 20 per cent of the range have developmental delay that should not be ignored. In Chapters 7, 8 and 10 a standardised data base is given. The tests described have been standardised on a sample of 425 children.* The standardised data base is given in graphical form, for considering an individual child's scores in terms of variation from the average, and for conversion of individual scores into age-level equivalents. The findings can be used as guidelines on the most appropriate action, *i.e.* for re-testing in a few weeks; therapy; investigation; or referral for detailed evaluation of children showing important deviations (Table 4.III).

*The standardisation sample (425 singletons aged 18 months to 4½ years) was drawn from the district birth registers in a South London health district (350), and from the computerised records of a market town in Wiltshire (75), using random number tables. These 425 children attending for the tests were 71 per cent and 90 per cent respectively of 578 originally selected. The sample excluded children on a 'handicapped' register, others with a known disability, those known to have suffered severe adverse social conditions including child abuse, those for whom English was not one of the languages used at home, and children of military personnel living on a military housing estate. 73 per cent were white, 22 per cent were black and 5 per cent were of Asian descent. The social class of the sample, using the Registrar General's classification, with figures for England and Wales 1981 in brackets, were: I and II, 26.2 per cent (31.5); III, 44.8 per cent (47.1); and IV and V, 29.0 per cent (21.5). The sample was used for standardisation of: (i) clinical tests of hearing according to age (see p. 39); (ii) bus puzzle and miniature toys for language development (see pp. 56 and 75); (iii) performance tests (p. 63) and (iv) vision test (p. 44).

5
CLINICAL TESTS OF HEARING

The introduction of clinical tests of hearing as a routine in child health centres at seven months has proved to be a landmark. It focused the attention of paediatricians, child health doctors and health visitors on the importance of looking more specifically at the development of young children. It gave parents a directive where to go for professional advice when they had worries about their child's progress. The interest of the press and media in developmental problems of young children has led to a wider public interest in development.

History
Important points are:
(1) parents' observations of an infant's auditory behaviour
(2) any history of deafness in the family
(3) any recent feverish illnesses, and
(4) an infant's experience of colds and respiratory infections.

Tests
The auditory response cradle is a micro-processor device used in some neonatal departments to detect congenital sensorineural deafness. Results appear promising. Recent major advances in the technology of hearing-aids has made it possible also to begin treatment at an early age and this, it is hoped, may improve the ability of severely deaf children to communicate in speech in adult life. Clinical testing remains necessary as some forms of congenital deafness do not become apparent until later in childhood; middle-ear infections are common even in the very young.

Six weeks to six months
Six to 15 weeks
Place the baby in supine. Shake a small clapper bell gently 15cm from the ear on the ear level.

In response, movements of the baby's limbs cease and the eyes open wide. If the baby is crying this ceases.

The test is a response to *sound* and does not necessarily imply a normal range of hearing. Absence of this response suggests a possible developmental problem or a hearing loss. Investigation by the audiology and/or paediatric department is indicated.

16 to 24 weeks
Place the baby in supine on a mattress.

Stroke the back of a spoon on the rim of a cup at 45cm from the baby's ear on his ear level. This is an interesting sound but is full of harmonics.

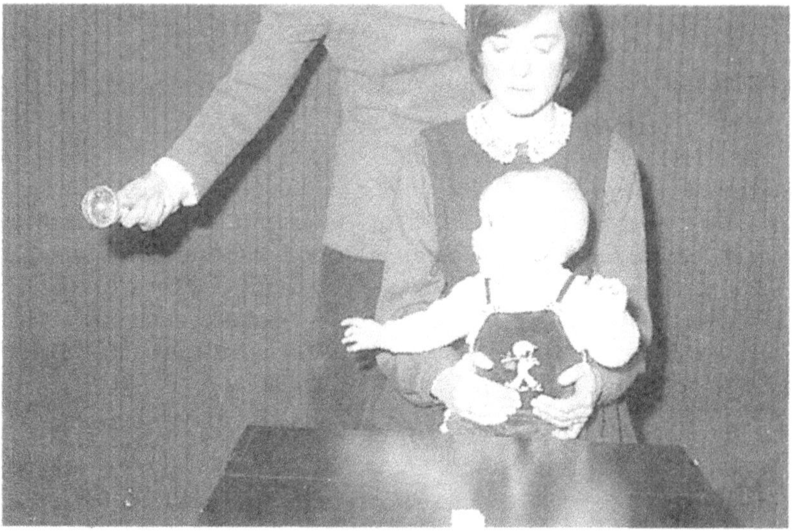

Fig. 5.1. Distraction test: Manchester rattle.

A normal response is head turning towards the side from which the sound comes without actual location of the sound source.

This test shows that the infant responds to sound, *i.e.* he has useful hearing, but does not necessarily indicate a normal range of hearing. Absence of a response suggests a developmental problem or hearing loss. Further investigation in a paediatric centre or audiology unit is indicated.

Seven months to 20 months

The infant is seated on mother's knee and supported upright. Two people are involved in testing: (i) the doctor or health visitor, responsible for directing and interpreting the results of the test, and (ii) the assistant who must be trained in the proper use of sound-making toys, and be aware of the necessity to avoid unnecessary movement, casting a shadow or wafting perfume.

Distraction test

CUP AND SPOON

Stroke the back of a spoon on the rim of a cup, taking care not to make a clunk as the spoon touches the rim. The sound has a wide range of frequencies and its validity is doubtful, but because it is a familiar sound, it is useful as a starter.

HIGH-FREQUENCY RATTLE TESTS

1. The Manchester rattle* is held horizontally at 1m from the ear on ear level and is rolled three or four times (Fig. 5.1).

*Obtainable from the Department of Audiology, University of Manchester, Manchester M13 9PL.

2. The Stycar rattle*, held vertically downwards 30cm from the ear on ear level, is used with a stirring motion repeated three or four times.

VOICE

The assistant should cover his mouth with his hand during all voice tests to prevent blowing on the ear.

'Ss-ss' is repeated three or four times; 'Oo-oo' is repeated three or four times. Then a short sentence is spoken, using the infant's name in a low voice (but not a whisper).

METHOD

Place yourself in front of the infant at a distance of 2m. The assistant stands behind the mother and child with sound-making toys ready to hand. Encourage the infant's attention by lightly using a toy, then put it out of sight as a signal to the assistant to give the sound stimulus. The sound-making objects are used in turn on each side of the infant's head.

A NORMAL RESPONSE

The infant turns his head and visually locates the source of the sound, equally on both sides.

If responses are absent or doubtful, the child should be referred to the audiology centre. If for any reason you are not sure of the results obtained, the child should be retested four weeks later.

Distraction tests are used for all children up to 20 months of age. Interpretation of results becomes more difficult from 13 to 20 months, because the infant at that age is no longer impelled to confirm visually what he has heard. The same stimulus should not be repeated consecutively on each side at this age, as the child may rapidly condition to the situation. In case of doubt a very low-voiced 'Would you like a sweetie?'† may produce a remarkable result.

20 months to 4½ years

The child is seated at a nursery table. The doctor places himself in front of the child near to his eye level. Children from 20 months of age upwards can normally be tested using co-operative tests involving language.

20 to 24 months

Larger-than-miniature toys test (Stycar*): five to seven toys are placed in a row on the table (cup, spoon, plane, fork, doll, knife and brick). Take care not to place the cutlery together, because young children tend to pick them up and 'bunch' them together in one hand.

Check that the child can select the toys correctly on verbal command.

*Obtainable from NFER, Darville House, 2 Oxford Street, East Windsor, Bucks SL4 1DF.

†'Sweetie' (candy) is universally understood by British children, and has the added advantage of being a high-frequency word!

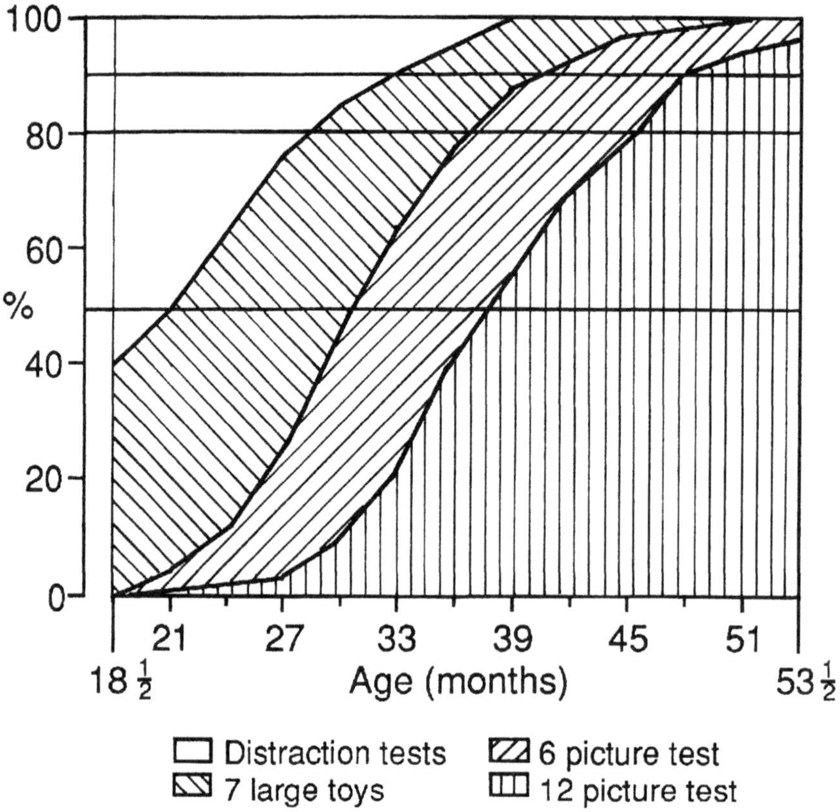

Fig. 5.2. Percentage of children able to achieve Stycar tests of hearing by age. *Diagonal lines, left:* percentage of children by age who can co-operate 7 large toy test but not yet the 6-picture or 12-picture test. *Diagonal lines, right:* percentage of children by age who can co-operate in 6-picture test but not yet the 12-picture test. *Vertical lines:* percentage of children by age who can co-operate in 12-picture test. (These figures are based on an unpublished study by Egan on a standardisation sample of 425 children—see p. 38.)

Remember that at this age the child's attention control is fixed on one object, so on each occasion you may have to take the toy gently from his hand and replace it on the table. Tell the child 'Now I am going to say it very quietly'. Move to a position at the side of the child so that your mouth (covered) is 45cm from the ear. This obviates the need to occlude the other ear provided that minimal voicing (*not* a whisper) is used. Name the toys in random order. Repeat the test on the other ear. Failure to select correctly suggests possible hearing loss.

SONKSEN LADYBIRD PICTURE TEST* (Sonksen 1985)

This test incorporates high- and low-frequency discriminations. It is more sensitive than the previous test and is therefore the test of choice as soon as the child is able

*Available from Wolfson Centre, Institute of Child Health, Mecklenburgh Square, London WC1N 2AP.

to select pictures (of a doll, a dog, a ball, a bath and a bus) correctly when named to him in a conversational voice. The technique is as described in the previous test. Failure to select any picture correctly suggests hearing loss.

MCCORMICK TOY DISCRIMINATION TEST (McCormick 1977)
This is an alternative test using a set of small toys: cup, duck, plate, plane, lamb, man, key, tree, shoe, spoon, house, horse and cow. The toys are placed on the table in front of the child. Check that the child recognises them by name, using a conversational voice. The technique is the same as in the two previous tests, and failure to select correctly suggests hearing loss.

STYCAR SIX-PICTURE TEST*
In this test there are six pictures (ship, pig, feet, seat, fish and chick) on a single card. Check that the child can select the pictures named to him in a conversational voice.

Move to a position 3m from the child at an angle of 45 degrees. Face him, cover the mouth, and using a carrier phrase ('Show me the ——') name the pictures at random. Do not whisper—just voice the names. Failure to select pictures correctly suggests a hearing loss, and reveals difference in hearing levels in each ear.

STYCAR 12-PICTURE TEST*
This test is similar to the six-picture test but there is a wider selection of named pictures which include more sophisticated phonemes for discrimination and a high vocabulary (key, tree, feet, seat, teeth, leaf, dish, fish, wheel, pig, chick and ship). The technique is as described above. It is important to avoid juxtaposition of names with similar sounds, *e.g.* fish and dish (Fig. 5.2).

Results
In each of the five tests described, failure to make correct naming of any picture or object suggests some degree of hearing loss which requires:
(1) examination with an auroscope for evidence of middle-ear infection
(2) referral to an audiology clinic for impedance tests or other investigation, or
(3) if in any doubt, follow-up in three months.

*Available from NFER, Darville House, 2 Oxford Street, East Windsor, Bucks SL4 1DF.

6

VISION—TESTS OF VISUAL BEHAVIOUR AND VISUAL ACUITY

Normal vision is dependent on:

(1) the physical properties of the transparent media, *i.e.* lens and cornea; the co-ordinated action of extra-ocular muscles, and the state of the retina

(2) the state of the optic nerves, optic chiasma and optic tract; lateral geniculate body; and the occipital cortex.

Vision is the dominant modality in the early years of life. It (i) promotes social communication, (ii) stimulates touch, reach and grasp, and encourages spatial recognition, (iii) influences the development of balancing reactions, (iv) reinforces auditory learning, and (v) contributes to the acquisition of language.

Poor vision puts constraints on all aspects of learning.

Visual perception—the ability to understand what is seen—develops at *near* distance in the early months of life. Refractive errors such as high hypermetropia and/or astigmatism adversely affect near and distant vision and may be present soon after birth (Table 6.I), and thus may hinder the infant's learning to a greater or lesser degree. Both conditions carry a high risk of strabismus and amblyopia. The hypermetropic or astigmatic eye requires a considerable degree of accommodation for near vision which leads to high risk of strabismus. Binocular vision may then not develop; suppression of the consequent double image may lead to amblyopia—a condition in which true central vision may be impaired and ultimately lost. Infants at the age of one year with a refractive error of +2.5D or more were found to be 20 times more likely to develop strabismus and amblyopia than children with more emmetropic vision (Ingram 1979).

A critical or sensitive period for the development of amblyopia has been shown to occur in kittens (Ikeda 1980).

Amblyopia causes reduced visual acuity in eyes that are organically healthy (Ingram 1980) and may occur even in the absence of a cosmetically detectable

TABLE 6.I

Acuity and accommodation in refractive anomalies (Gardiner 1982)

Anomaly	*Accommodation required*		*Effect on visual acuity*	
	Near	*Distance*	*Near*	*Distance*
High hypermetropia	++	+	Impaired	Impaired
Moderate hypermetropia	+	±	Impaired	Normal
Astigmatism	+	Nil*	Impaired	Impaired
Myopia	±	Nil	Normal	Impaired

Reproduced by kind permission of P. A. Gardiner and MTP Press Ltd.
*Unless combined with hypermetropia.

squint. The condition is irreversible after seven years of age. Some ophthalmologists doubt the efficacy of occlusion therapy after the fifth birthday. The new rotatory gratings treatment using black-and-white patterned cards has had some success but requires considerable concentration by the child. The treatment does not improve non-strabismus amblyopia.

Ingram (1980) found that 75 per cent of children identified as having amblyopia had no cosmetically detectable squint; 70 per cent were missed until school age, and 50 per cent of children with strabismus were not diagnosed before school entry. Can we identify infants and young children who have reduced visual acuity, or who require further investigation by an ophthalmologist because they are at risk of developing amblyopia? Screening of young infants in the first year by photo-refraction (Atkinson *et al.* 1984) is one approach which is being studied. It requires expensive equipment and a back-up team.

Can we rely on parents to suspect poor vision?

Parents do observe some aspects of unusual behaviour in very young infants—the neonate who does not look at mother when feeding always engenders anxiety. Unusual movements of the eyes or a white patch in the pupil may be seen. These are all important observations requiring investigation. If parental suspicion is confirmed, immediate expert opinion should be sought. On the whole parents are better than professionals in suspecting squint, although occasionally they may be deceived by a wide nasal ridge. Diagnosis depends on a cover test.

Parents do *not* appear to suspect moderate problems of poor vision in early childhood. The child himself does not complain but appears to accept his poor vision as normal. There are countless stories of children who at the age of seven or eight years suddenly found how different their world actually looked when at last their refractive error was diagnosed at a routine vision test at school.

Examination

History

Mother's view of her young infant's visual behaviour is always important. She may be helped by questions such as 'Does he watch the cat or birds?' and 'Does he sit close to the TV screen and return there even when moved back?'

A strong family history of hypermetropia, squint and amblyopia in parents and siblings is important, as is a parental history of myopia. Age of onset of myopia is variable in families and is generally later in childhood.

Six weeks to six months

Place the baby in supine on a mattress and observe the appearance of the eyes.

Pupil reactions

Use a pen torch held 5 to 7cm from each eye in turn. Look for brisk contraction of pupils.

Note: reflected light in the centre of each pupil is not a reliable test for squint, because the reflection may be eccentric even in normal eyes.

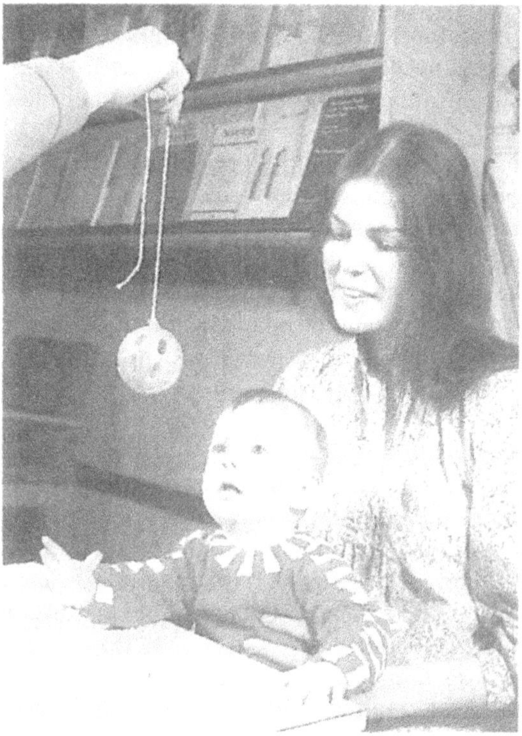

Fig. 6.1. Visual following.

Red reflex

Hold the ophthalmoscope 35cm from each of the baby's eyes in turn. The reflected light should be uniformly *red*. Any break-up of the clear red requires immediate investigation by an ophthalmologist because this may be indicative of cataract, retinoblastoma or other severe ophthalmic pathology.

Visual fixation and visual following

SIX WEEKS

Lean down over the baby to some 30cm from his face and talk gently until he fixes his eyes on yours. Then *immediately cease all sound* and move your head slowly to each side to induce following and full abduction of the infant's eyes. Look for nystagmus.

INFANTS 16 TO 24 WEEKS

Hold a spinning ball suspended on a string at some 30 to 35cm from the baby's face to induce visual fixation. Then move the ball slowly, first to one side then the other, to induce full abduction. The normal baby will visually follow the ball. Look for nystagmus.

Poor visual fixation and/or visual following are significant and suggest a severe developmental problem such as mental handicap or poor vision. Referral for paediatric opinion is probably the action of choice.

Six months to 20 months

The infant is seated supported upright on mother's lap. Look for pupil reactions using a pencil torch. Reactions should be brisk.

Visual fixation and visual following

Stand in front of the infant and attract his gaze with a spinning ball suspended on a string. Move the ball slowly to one side until full abduction of the eyes is seen—usually when you have reached a point almost behind mother's head (Fig. 6.1).

Note: this test cannot be carried out if you are seated in your chair!

Repeat this manoeuvre to the opposite side.

Poor fixation and/or poor visual following suggest a severe developmental problem, handicap or poor vision problem. Failure to achieve full abduction of one eye suggests strabismus.

Cover test

A cover test is an essential part of every vision test. It can be carried out at any age.

Position yourself in front of the child holding a small movable toy as a lure and verbally encourage the child to look at it. Remember that a pencil or finger is not sufficiently interesting. Do not be tempted to put your hand on the infant's head and use your thumb as the cover. Touching the head is commonly fiercely resented by young children. The thumb is in any case an ineffective cover. Remember that the range of peripheral vision is wide.

A card can be used as cover, or you may use your hand. If the hand is used it should be held pointing downwards, wrist fully flexed and fingers extended and held close together. A flick of the wrist allows rapid repetition of cover/uncover procedure.

Young babies tend to look first at the cover but gaze can be attracted and held by a movable lure.

Talk to the child to encourage him to hold his gaze on the toy: 'Look at my doggie! Watch his tail (ear, eye)'. As soon as fixation is attained, cover the infant's right eye and look at his left eye. There should be *no* movement of the left eye to take up fixation.

If the left eye moves *out* to take up fixation, there is a left convergent squint.

If the left eye moves *in* to take up fixation, there is a left divergent squint.

The cover is then removed from the right eye which should maintain its position. If the right eye moves, a latent squint may be present. The cover test is then repeated on the right eye.

A suspected squint should *always* be referred immediately to an ophthalmological department.

The Sonksen picture test

Sonksen and Macrae (1987) found that realistic coloured pictures of familiar objects from the Ladybird picture books are seen clearly from a distance of 3m by children with 3/3 vision. Children with induced refractive errors and vision of 3/4.5

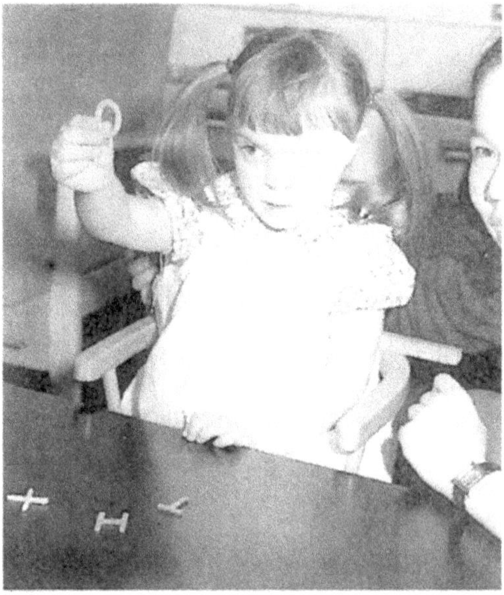

Fig. 6.2. Visual acuity test. Matching with plastic letters; occlusion with Dermicel patch.

or 3/6 had difficulty with some pictures (Grade III visual complexity). Pictures from this grade are currently being evaluated as a vision test to identify children in the age-range 20 months to five years with minor to major defects of acuity.

The test is quick, easy to administer and has promise as a screening tool.

MATERIAL

Eight coloured pictures of familiar objects include two training pictures (car and shoe) and six test pictures (sweets, brush/comb, chocolate, bicycle, orange and buttons).

METHOD

The child is seated at a nursery table. Show him the two training pictures in turn, asking: 'What is it?'

This is not a language test so any gesture or reply which shows that the picture is correctly identified is acceptable, *e.g.* 'brum-brum' for car, or 'marties'* for sweets.

Move to a measured distance of 3m and show the six test pictures in turn asking 'What is it?' If the child gives a wrong answer, come forward and give the picture to him. If he identifies it, his failure at 3m is visual. A fine visual discrimination is required to see, for example, the holes in the buttons which differentiates them from other round objects. A child who has difficulty in visual discrimination of any one picture should be referred for further visual examination to an ophthalmology department.

*Meaning 'Smarties', brightly coloured sweets or candy.

Visual acuity

There are two major requirements for the examination of visual acuity:

(1) a child must be able to co-operate in a test comparable to the adult model, *i.e.* to match letters in a linear chart of standard Snellen letters at a distance of 6m, and

(2) the child must be willing to accept occlusion so that each eye is tested separately.

Plastic letters for matching (Fig. 6.2)

Experience has shown that young children under 42 months of age quickly become bored with the task of pointing to letters on a key card and so to pay sustained attention at 6m. Egan and Brown (1984*a*) found that a child's interest could be held if plastic letters* (designed on the basis of a square) were used for matching. The letters can be picked up and waved triumphantly and the task becomes an interesting game. The percentage of children at 33 months of age able to co-operate in an adult-type test increased from 38 to 65 per cent—a very substantial gain.

Linear chart for testing distant visual acuity

The Sheridan/Gardiner linear chart is today widely used in nursery and primary schools and in health centres for testing visual acuity of children in the age-range three to seven years. Two features in design seriously restrict its value: the bottom line of the chart defines normal distant visual acuity 6.6. The choice of only four letters, 'H', 'A', 'O' and 'V' makes interpretations of findings difficult. 'O' is identifed very early by preschool children, but 'A' and 'V' are commonly confused because of a characteristic tendency in these young chidren to reverse shapes. In effect this reduces choice to two letters 'H' and 'O'.

Detection of amblyopia depends on the crowding effect presented by a line of letters in which spacing between each letter is the same as the width of the Snellen square of the letter itself. The amblyopic eye may see the first letter of any line. In this chart, spacing between letters is very considerably wider so that the crowding effect is lost. Single optotype should never be used for testing vision at primary-care level.

Visual acuity test using Egan/Calver linear chart and plastic letters

The Egan/Calver linear chart† has been designed in the paediatric/ophthalmology department, Guy's Hospital, to overcome these difficulties. Great care has been taken to equalise spacing of letters to the size of Snellen square letters of each line. 'A', which young children commonly confuse with 'V', has been replaced by 'L'. A slide marker is used to define the line being tested. Point to the 60 letter; then to the 24 and 18 or 12 lines, taking the letters right across the line.

*Plastic letters available from the Test Agency, Cournswood House, North Dean, High Wycombe, Bucks HP14 4NW.

†Egan/Calver Linear Chart available from Davis Keeler Ltd, Clewer Hill Road, Windsor, Berks SL4 4AA.

Say 'Now let's find these tiny ones', indicating letters across the line of size 6 letters. If the child is not able to match *every* letter on the 6 line, take him along the line of size 9 letters, and so on until a whole line is completed correctly.

Remember that children with an amblyopic eye may successfully read the first or last letter of a line. Repeat test with each eye separately.

Occlusion

Many different types of occluder have been tried over the years. The author, in a paediatric/ophthalmology clinic found that the acceptance rate of a Dermicel patch by infants from six to 13 or 14 months is high (over 90 per cent). The patch is translucent and is probably less frightening to an infant than other occluders which put one eye in the dark. Occlusion of the eye is not well accepted by children of 24 to 33 months. In the standardisation sample only 25 per cent were occluded successfully. The acceptance rate rose slowly to 40 per cent at 33 months, then increased rapidly to 80 per cent by 39 months (Egan and Brown 1984*a*).

Dermicel patch

A square patch is readily torn from the roll. The square is held diagonally and one corner applied to the bridge of the nose. A quick sweep of the hand leaves the patch *in situ*. When the test has been completed the patch should be removed first from the bridge of the nose to avoid any pull on the eyelashes.

Near vision

The 'hundreds and thousands'* test is used for observing near vision of infants of six to 20 months. A sweet is released at some point during a sweep of the examiner's hand across the table (Sonksen 1979). It shows visual awareness of the objects but is not a measure of visual acuity (Baird and Hall 1985). Failure to see these sweets suggests poor vision or other developmental problem.

Once a child can co-operate in an adult-type test, *i.e.* matching letters to a linear chart of standard Snellen letters at 6m, near vision can be tested when appropriate by matching letters to a Reduced Snellen Chart, or to the Sonksen/Silver acuity system—near card. Near vision need not be tested routinely if distant vision is normal.

The Sonksen/Silver acuity system†

The Sonksen/Silver acuity system (Sonksen and Silver 1988) provides an accurate measure of distant and near acuity using Snellen 6m standard specifications. The test, like the Egan/Calver test, can be achieved by most children from 3½ years of age.

The system is provided in two forms: (i) screening pack, and (ii) pack for specialist/diagnostic setting.

*'Hundreds and thousands': pinhead-sized, brightly coloured sweets (candy) used for cake decoration.

†Sonksen/Silver acuity system available from Davis Keeler Ltd, Clewer Hill Road, Windsor, Berks SL4 4AA.

SCREENING PACK

Training booklet and key card. The latter has six 45cm letters arranged in a widely spaced crescent.

Booklet 18–3 has one line of five letters, each of size 18, 12, 9 and 4.5m, and two lines of five letters each of size 6 and 3m.

The near card has 10 lines each of five letters, N48 to N4.5 equivalent. There is also a black plastic pointer.

DISTANCE ACUITY

Sit the child at a nursery table with the key card for matching. Make sure that the child can match letters by using the training booklet and key card at reading distance. The booklet has been designed for use in testing visual acuity at 3m or 6m. This must be measured accurately.

At 3m (the commonly available distance in child health clinics or GP surgeries), using the booklet, point to the first letter of the 18 line using the black pointer upright under the letter. Repeat down to the 3 line. If all five letters are not correctly matched, return to the next largest size line and repeat along the whole line.

The smallest display in which all five letters are correctly matched gives the measure of acuity.

The test is then repeated for each eye using occlusion.

If the test is carried out at 3m and the child matches all the letters in the 3 line, the result is recorded as 3/3. The result should *not* be converted into 6m equivalents.

GUIDANCE FOR ACTION

Children with visual acuity of 3/6 or worse in either eye should be referred to an eye clinic.

Children with one line difference between the eyes and acuity of 3/4.5 in the worse eye should be retested in two to three months and then annually.

Children with *equal* acuity in each eye which is 3/4.5 or better should have routine checks.

NEAR VISION

Near vision can be tested, if required, using the key card, near card and black pointer.

The technique is similar. Use the black pointer to point to the first letter of each line down to the N4.5 line, then point to each of the five letters in that line. If all five letters are not correctly identified, return to the previous line. Measure of near acuity is the smallest display for which all five letters are correctly matched from a distance of 25cm.

7
TESTS FOR EARLY LANGUAGE SKILLS

Early development of language skills becomes evident as understanding of gesture, situation, simple words and, ultimately, of sentences.

Comprehension is the cognitive factor in development and is expected to advance steadily with age. Comprehension may be shown by gesture or actions without necessarily the use of expressive speech.

Expressive language on the other hand may progress in a more individual way, and within normal limits at varying rates. Some infants, though not all, acquire a naming vocabulary by stages, *i.e.* through the use of a generic term, and a little later a functional term, before the proper name is used. Progress in speech development may appear to slow down during a period when other executive skills such as learning to walk or to climb are advancing rapidly. Parents after such a period not uncommonly express surprise that their child seems to make a sudden leap forward in understanding: 'I didn't know he knew that!'.

From 20 months a child is expected to join words to express ideas. Acquisition of grammar during the following year may be variable. Consonant substitutions and difficulties with double sounds are common.

A child of three years is expected to be intelligible within his own family. Motivation to make a sentence with a verb may depend on whether it is possible to convey meaning by a simpler form of expression.

A four-year-old is normally grammatical. Nouns, verbs, adjectives, adverbs and other parts of speech are used correctly.

Comprehension and expressive language should always be tested separately.

History

History is always important: *i.e.* a family history of deviant development of language skills; mental handicap; deafness; late talking; articulation problems or stammering in the family. (Stammering in young children under five years of age is almost always due to hesitancy associated with the development of expressive speech and is best ignored; at most, recommend a helpful word.)

A social history may reveal adverse home conditions leading to serious deprivation of input. This can result in a general lowering of the language base.

Specific developmental language disorder in the family as a primary constitutional disorder carries a high recurrence rate in males (Sonksen 1979).

Six weeks to six months

Your objective during this period is to establish that social communication with the mother is developing.

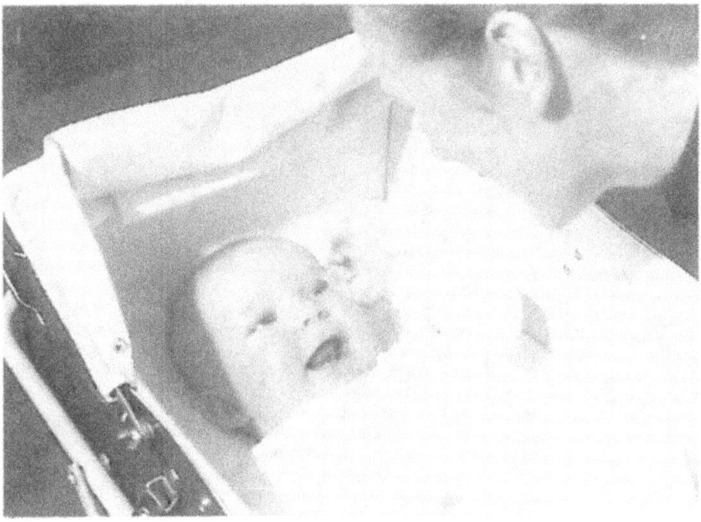

Fig. 7.1. Responsive vocalisations at 20 weeks.

Six weeks

Evidence may stem largely from questions to mother:

(1) Does the baby look at mother when feeding? Absence of eye-to-eye contact suggests serious developmental problems.

(2) Does the baby smile back? Absence of smiling back at eight or nine weeks suggests serious developmental delay.

(3) Does the baby recognise mother's voice and is he soothed by it? Absence suggests congenital hearing loss or developmental problems.

20 weeks

Lean over the baby and talk to him (Fig. 7.1). Does he vocalise responsively? This is a manifestation of 'taking turns'.

(Always allow for preterm birth.)

Six months to 20 months

The baby is seated supported on mother's lap at a small table of convenient height so that he can look down on toys placed there.

'Give me' test, 10 months

Put a cube into the baby's hand. Ask mother what form of words she uses when playing this game: 'Ta', 'Give it to me', 'Can I have it?'

Hold out your palm and use the appropriate phrase. Does the infant offer the cube to your hand? Failure to understand your gesture and simple words by 12 months suggests delay in comprehension.

Pointing, 12 months

Ask mother: 'How does he let you know what he wants?'

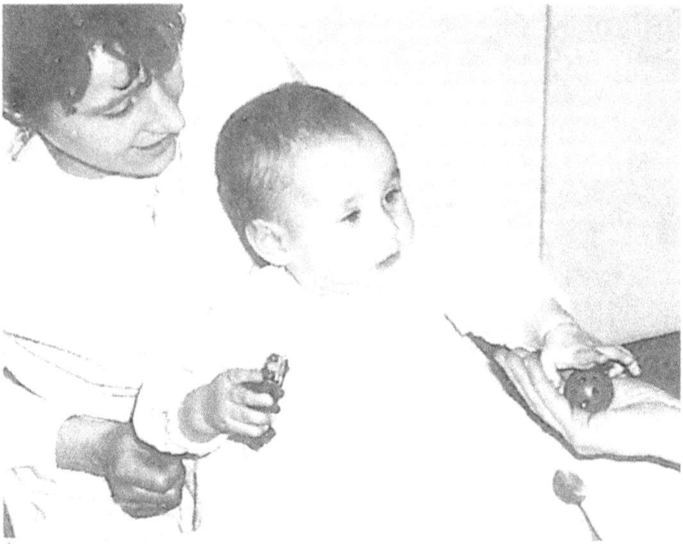

Fig. 7.2. Handing toys on request by name at 14 months.

The pointing gesture at this age is a developmental landmark. Its absence in the following months is significant and suggests delay. On the other hand, if a child in the 13- to 20-month age-group is proving unco-operative, observation of the pointing gesture may be reassuring to the assessor that progress is probably within normal limits. Follow-up examination in two or three months is advisable.

Expressive language

You will almost certainly have to rely on mother's report of sounds made by the infant in the first 13 months.

6 months: does he make double sounds—*e.g.* 'dad-dad'?

9 months: does he babble in strings, *e.g.* 'dad-dad-dad-dad'?

10 to 12 months: does the infant practise a series of sounds? Parents often report that 'He says everything—dad, mum, bath, nan.' This is imitative babble, *not* yet use of words with meaning. At times the sound may appear appropriate to the situation. Parents' immediate pleasure is strong encouragement to the infant.

Absence of this sequence of sound-making may suggest hearing loss or developmental delay.

13 to 20 months

Encourage the child of 13 months to sit at a nursery table rather than on mother's lap.

The tests are designed to reveal the development of the following skills:

(1) symbolic play—self-related from 13 months; detached-from-self (doll-orientated) at 18 to 20 months
(2) comprehension of names of familiar objects from 14 months
(3) expressive language (naming of familiar objects) from 15 months.

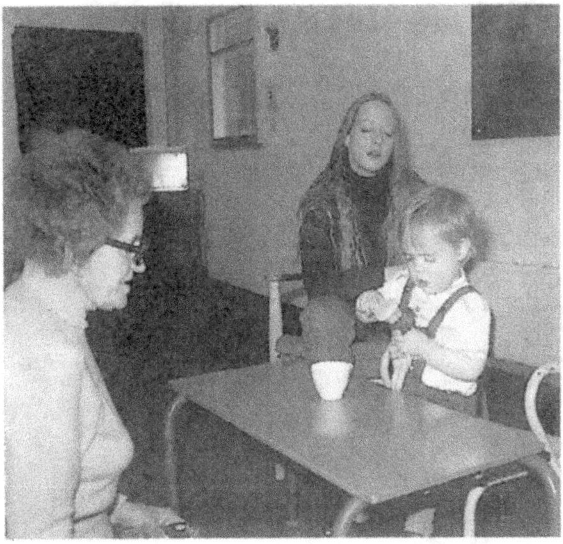

Fig. 7.3. Detached-from-self play at 18 months.

MATERIALS

Cup, spoon, hairbrush, doll and toy aeroplane.

TEST

Comprehension: seat yourself in front of the child with the toys concealed from view. Offer each toy in turn, asking 'What is it?' Repeat the question several times. Attention of a child in this age-range tends to be fixed on an object of his choice, and he may not be willing to part with it. Take each toy gently from his hand and put it out of sight momentarily while offering him the next. Does the child of 13 months use one of the toys appropriately in self-related play, *e.g.* drinking from the cup, brushing his hair, or feeding himself with the spoon?

14 to 15 months: replace the objects on the table. Hold out your hand, palm upwards 'Give me the —' naming each in turn in random order (Fig. 7.2).

Take care not to eye-point the object named, or indicate it by the position of your hand.

Replace each object before naming another so as to maintain a choice.

A child between 14 and 18 months is expected to select correctly one or two objects named to him. He may select all five correctly from 18 months. Thus comprehension may be shown without a child necessarily speaking.

Does the child from 18 months show detached-from-self play with any of the toys, *e.g.* feeding the doll with cup or spoon, or brushing the doll's hair? (Fig. 7.3).

Expressive language: when asked 'What is it?' (see above), a child of 13 to 15 months may jargon excitedly. He is expected to name one or two from 15 months and four to six from 18 months.

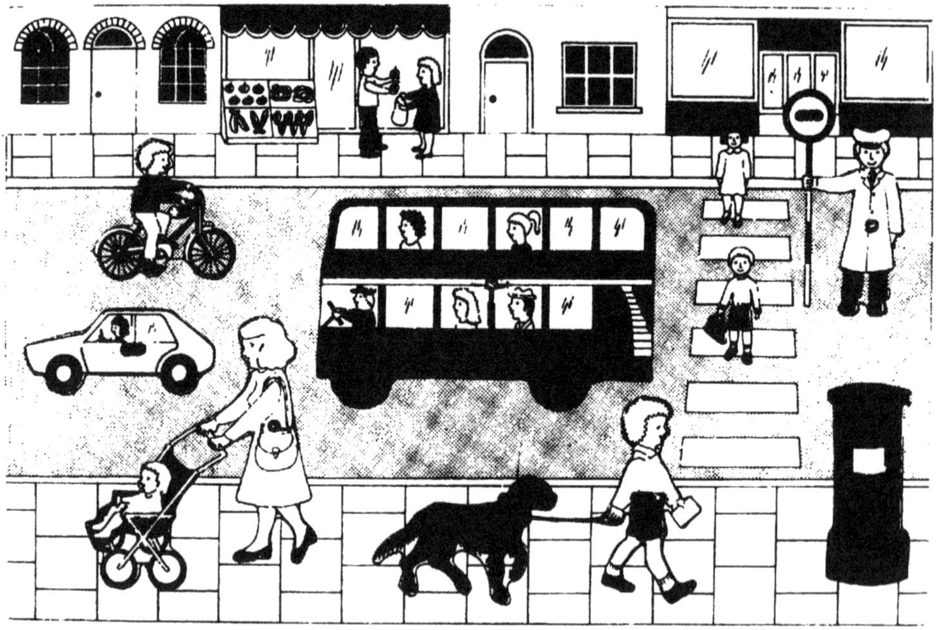

Fig. 7.4. Egan bus puzzle test (from Egan and Brown 1984*b*). (Red double-decker buses and post-boxes are not necessarily familiar worldwide! However the child's interpretation of a salient feature of each is being tested here.)

Interpretation of findings

This requires considerable clinical judgement because reversion to earlier patterns of behaviour is not uncommon. A single instance of self-related play by a child under 18 months suggests there is little cause for anxiety; any doll-oriented play at 18 months is reassuring. Absence of expected levels of symbolic play is significant and requires follow-up and investigation.

Delay in comprehension cannot be ignored. Investigation by a paediatrician, speech therapist and/or audiologist should be considered.

Expressive delay with normal comprehension requires mother's report of words used at home. Management of the child to date may be relevant, for example a demanding older sibling may limit mother's availability to talk with and or read to him, or social conditions in the home may be adverse.

Clinical tests of hearing are essential in every case of suspected language delay.

Allowance should be made for preterm birth in the first 15 months. Delay after that age is an indication for further follow-up.

20 months to 4½ years

*The Egan bus puzzle test of developing language skills** (Fig. 7.4)

The test has been designed to determine whether language development of children

*Obtainable as a full kit from the Test Agency, Cournswood House, North Dean, High Wycombe, Bucks HP14 4NW.

in the age-range 20 months to 4½ years is progressing as expected. It reveals the broad pattern of a child's understanding of words and situations, his ability to convey this by gesture or words, and it provides a profile of any discrepancies within these areas.

The test is not intended for the analysis of language disorders. It is unlikely that primary-care doctors will have the time or training for a task which needs the psycholinguistic skills of the speech therapist.

The test offers a standardised data base in comprehension and expressive language for converting individual children's scores into age equivalents, and considering them in terms of variation from the average. The data base is given in graphical forms. The findings can be used as guidelines on the most appropriate referral for detailed evaluation of children showing important deviations.

Age-range

20 months to four years. The ceiling is then reached for normal children but the test is also useful for older children who function within the age-range of the test.

TIME

The test can be completed in eight minutes.

MATERIAL

A wooden inset puzzle depicts a brightly coloured street scene with nine lift-out pieces (dog, car, bus, postbox, buggy with baby, mummy pushing buggy, boy on bicycle, boy with letter leading dog and 'lollipop man' at street-crossing). Each piece is readily removed by a small knob at the centre.

The puzzle is instantly attractive to children and provokes spontaneous talk as well as social communication.

PURPOSE

Developing language skills: expressive verbal labels, naming the pieces of the puzzle; comprehension of verbal labels, correct choosing of the pieces named by the proper name; comprehension of six questions on situations illustrated; expressive language—responses to six questions on situations illustrated; and intuitive thinking—naming unseen objects likely to be in mother's handbag.

Performance skills: recognition of shape, *i.e.* of the outline image in the tray; and orientation of pieces, *i.e.* applying the pieces correctly to the recess.

There are several general points to be observed in giving the test.

1. Talk to young children in simple words that you expect them to understand. For example, do not ask a two-year-old 'What is it called?' Mother would say 'What is it?'

2. Use repetition and demand freely, to avoid awkward silences. Give praise and encouragement. Never say 'no'. The child should not be allowed to experience a sense of failure. If he does not respond, or gives a wrong answer after two

TABLE 7.I

Examples of expressive verbal labels

Piece	*Scores 1*	*Scores 2*	*Scores 3*
Dog	Cat, horse, bow-wow	—	Dog
Car	Brum-brum	—	Car
Bus	Car, lorry	Train	Bus
Postbox	Door	Post office, phone-box	Letter-box, postbox
Buggy	Baby	—	Buggy, pram, push-chair
Lollipop man	Man, daddy	Milkman, postman, policeman	Lollipop man, crossing man, traffic man
Mummy	—	Lady	Mummy
Boy	—	—	Boy, girl
Bicycle	—	—	Bike, motorbike

chances, say what the correct answer is before going on to the next question.

3. Keep in mind the level of attention control to be expected of a child at his age-level. Remember that a child under 33 months cannot readily detach from the task to listen to a verbal instruction. Place your hands gently over his, then look him in the eye, give your instruction slowly and clearly, then release the hands to allow the task to be carried out.

Adhere to the instructions exactly as given for each section. Record raw scores concurrently, and compare total for each of six sections with data base provided in graphs.

METHOD

The test is arranged in four sections:

(1) expressive verbal labels (EVL)
(2) comprehension verbal labels (CVL), and performance skills—recognition of shape and orientation of pieces
(3) comprehension of six questions on situations illustrated; and expressive language, responses to questions, and
(4) objects likely to be present in Mummy's handbag (optional).

The assessor records raw score as a series of ticks in the appropriate boxes on the scoring sheet.

TEST

The child is seated at a nursery table with mother close by.

EXPRESSIVE VERBAL LABELS (Table 7.I)

Method: point to the dog and ask 'What is it?'

If the child tells you correctly, ask him to take the piece out and put it on the table, indicating the child's left-hand side of the tray. (This is important in the observation later of performance skills—see section 2.)

If necessary repeat 'What is it?' to give him a second chance. If he does not know, tell him and ask him to take the piece out.

Repeat with each piece until all nine are out on the table.

Generic term: a child may name the dog as 'cat' or 'horse'. He is telling you it is an animal, *i.e.* using a generic term.

Functional term: the lollipop man may be named 'milkman' or 'policeman'. The child is trying to express his understanding by giving the man a function.

Proper name: some children use the proper name from the beginning.

The scoring system takes account of these developing levels of maturity, by giving credit for early meaningful attempts by the younger age-groups, or recording persistence of immature terms by older children.

A tick is put in the appropriate box on the scoring sheet: generic term scores = 1, functional term scores = 2, and proper name scores = 3. The total score for EVLS is 27.

A table of some alternatives given by children in the standardisation sample is given opposite. The list is not intended to be exclusive.

COMPREHENSION OF VERBAL LABELS AND RECOGNITION OF SHAPE AND ORIENTATION OF PIECES

Method: ask the child to replace each piece named to him in turn.

Use the proper name, not the child's version of it, and take care not to eye-point the piece when naming it.

If the child makes a wrong choice, take the piece from him, replace it on the table and repeat your request, thus giving him a second chance. If he fails, select the correct piece for him and tell him to put it back. In these circumstances there is no score for CVL for that piece.

Recognition of shape is observed concurrently for each piece. It is useful to name pieces on the right-hand side of the board, *i.e.* 'postbox' and 'lollipop man' among the early selections, and to note whether the child's hand moves towards that side of the board before he has fully turned his head; showing that he has taken in the whole layout. This cannot be scored numerically but is a useful developmental marker.

Orientation of each piece to the recess can also be observed. Some experimentation is permissible by the under-threes.

Notes: 'Car', 'dog', 'bus' and 'baby' were understood earliest in the standardisation. It is wise to begin with one or two of these pieces when assessing younger groups.

When selecting the appropriate recess a child may aid his thinking by talking to himself: 'Where it go?' This is an intelligent response.

Total score for each part of this section is 9.

SECTION 3

A new approach in the thinking of the child will be required of him in order to show understanding of six questions on situations illustrated in the puzzle.

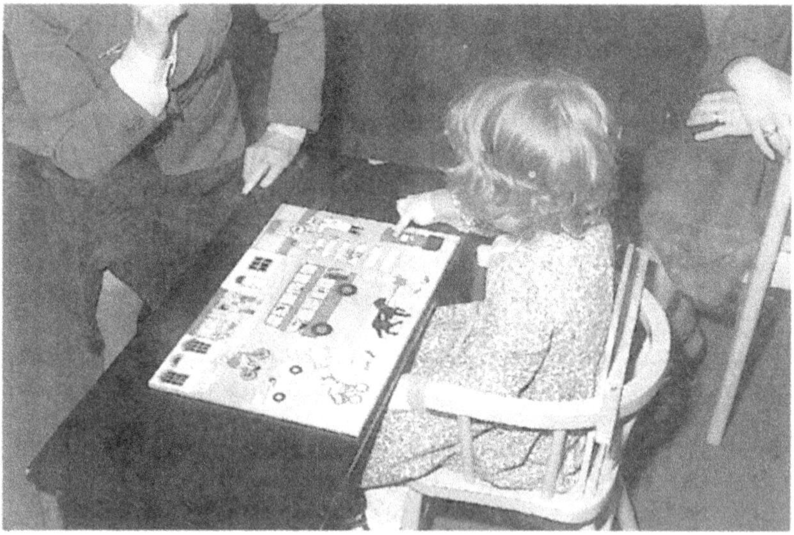

Fig. 7.5. 'What is the boy going to do with the letter?'

QUESTIONS

1. Q. Why do we have steps on the bus—what are they for?
   A. To go up top.
2. Q. What is Mummy doing?
   A. Pushing the buggy.
3. Q. What is she going to do with it? (letter)
   A. Put it in the postbox.
4. Q. What is he doing with his other hand?
   A. Walking the dog.
5. Q. What is this boy doing?
   A. Riding his bike.
6. Q. What is the lollipop man doing?
   A. Stopping the cars to let the children cross.

First draw the child's attention to the bus. 'Let's look at the bus. Show me the driver of the bus'. This is not scored, though 46 per cent of children at 30 months and 80 per cent at 39 months in the standardisation sample indicated the driver correctly.

COMPREHENSION

As each of the six questions is put to the child, indicate the part of the picture under discussion, but do *not* point to the action.

Give the six questions in the order presented.

Q1 is preceded by 'What are these?' pointing to the stairs (do not sweep your finger up and down!). This is introductory and is not scored. If the child does not reply, tell him. 'Why do we have steps on the bus?' 'What are steps (stairs) for?' The

repeat queston in its simpler form is for the under-threes. Use the first version when repeating the question for the over-threes.
Q2: 'What is Mummy doing?' Do not point to her hands on the buggy; point to her head. 'Baby' is not acceptable. Understanding is shown as 'push', 'pushing', 'pushing the buggy', 'taking the baby shopping'.
Q3. 'What is the boy going to do with the letter?' (Fig. 7.5). The question is introduced by pointing to the letter and asking 'What is it?' The answer is not scored. Common responses are 'purse', 'card', 'piece of paper'. Encourage the child by telling him 'I call it a letter. Shall we call it a letter?' Then ask Q3.
Q4. 'What is he doing with his other hand?' Point to the boy's shoulder, not to the hand in which he holds the letter; nor to the lead of the dog.
Q5. 'What is this boy doing?' Point to the boy's head, not the bike.
Q6. 'What is the lollipop man doing?' Point to the lollipop man's head. This question is expected to be beyond the experience of the youngest age-groups—under 2½ years. The earliest evidence of understanding by age is when the child points to the 'lollipop' itself and says 'stand' or 'hold' or 'cars'. This response is interpreted as awareness that the 'lollipop' has something to do with the man's function. It appears on average at 2½ years.

Part 2
Comprehension of questions is shown by any response whether by gesture or word(s) which reveals that the situation illustrated is understood.

There is a score of one for each correct response. *Maximum 6.*

Expressive language is scored concurrently as each question is put. A graded score not only helps the assessor to listen carefully to the child's actual responses but is one way to observe a child's grasp of grammar which is a learned process.

Replies to questions must relate to the situations illustrated. It is not simply a matter of counting words.

Gesture or single word—score 1; two or three words without a verb, or present participle only—score 2; three or more words including a verb—score 3. *Maximum score 18.*

Note: the reply must relate to the situation illustrated and convey the idea given in parentheses. For example, in Q1 ('Why do we have steps on the bus—What are steps for?') the reply "Cos we do' is a situational phrase repeated to cover lack of understanding. (Score 0.)

Or in Q6 ('What is the lollipop man doing?') the reply 'Gives you sweets and lollipops' is a play on words. (Score 0.)

If score for comprehension is 0 there cannot be a score for expressive language.

Articulation is noted but not scored. Remember that consonant substitution and difficulties with double consonants are normal until three years of age.

INTERPRETATION OF RESULTS
Graphs—EVLS; CVLS; recognition of shape; orientation; sentences understood and sentence (expressive) scores.

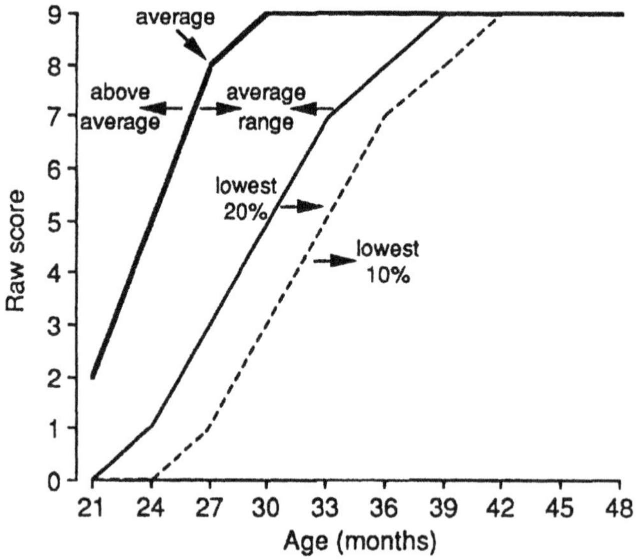

Fig. 7.6. The maximum number of pieces identified by at least 50, 80 and 90 per cent.

Six graphs are provided, one for each section of the test (for CVL, see Fig. 7.26). Raw scores are shown on the vertical axis. Age-groups each covering a three-month age-period designated by the mid-month of the group are on the horizontal axis.

Three curves are shown, each giving the score obtained by 50, 80 and 90 per cent of children in the standardisation sample.

Variation from the average. The child's age-group and total raw score are identified. If the point of intersection falls (i) on the 50 per cent curve, the child's score is average; and (ii) in the area on the *right* of the 50 per cent curve up to and including the 80 per cent curve, the child is scoring *in the average range*; (iii) in the area to the *right* of the 80 per cent curve, the child is scoring in the lowest 20 per cent; (iv) in the area to the *right* of the 90 per cent curve, the child's score is in the lowest 10 per cent.

Scores to the *left* of the 50 per cent curve are above average.

Thus, scores falling into group (iii) and (iv) identify those children for whom the doctor will wish to consider action to be taken.

The six graphs in the full list are designed on a grid so that the score related to age can be immediately pinpointed.

GUIDANCE FOR ACTION

The test identifies children whose scores are in the lowest 20 per cent as those who require further follow-up and investigation (see p. 38). Repeat hearing tests or referral to an audiology centre will be essential. Referral to a speech therapist or other specialist advice may often be required.

Specialist advice is likely to be seen as essential for children whose skills are those of the lowest 10 per cent.

8
DEVELOPMENTAL EXAMINATION OF PERFORMANCE SKILLS

The neonate has a primitive grasp with fingers and toes. This passes off between 12 and 16 weeks when learned skills such as reaching, precise grasp and release from the hand are developed. Early in the second year visuomotor skills require a child to 'see' the construction.

History
This includes history of pregnancy, labour and the puerperium; history of suspected motor disorder; and family history of late reading or poor writing.

Six weeks to six months
Six weeks
Note the flexed posture of the hands as the body lies in supine. Put a rattle into the baby's hand and observe that it is gripped firmly. Press the sole of the foot at the base of the toes and note flexion.

16 weeks
Put the baby in supine on a mattress. Hold a ball suspended on a string at 30cm from the baby's face. Does he try to reach it? Does he persist even as it rolls round his hand?

22 weeks
Sit the baby supported upright on mother's lap at a table on which one or two coloured 2.5cm cubes have been placed. Does he immediately make uncoordinated movements with his hands, palms downwards and fingers spread, in sustained attempts to reach them?

A delay of two or three weeks suggests a developmental problem or vision impairment.

24 weeks
Sit the baby on mother's lap supported upright at a table on which two cubes have been placed. Does he immediately reach for one, patting with the flat of his hand then scooping it up in a palmar grasp using four fingers but not the thumb to take one to his mouth? Does he do this with either hand?

Seven months to 20 months
Does he transfer the cube from one hand to the other?

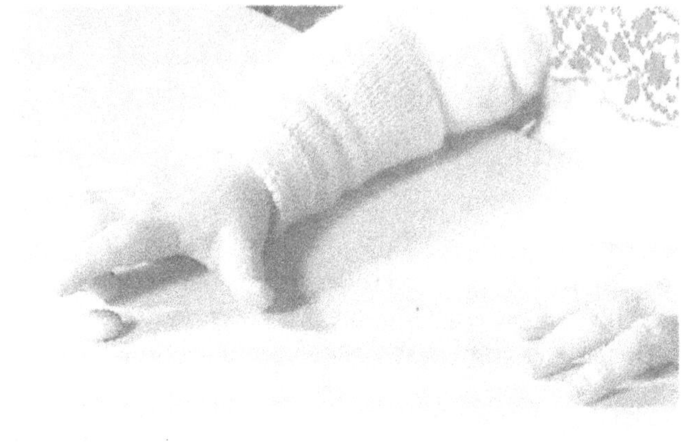

Fig. 8.1. Exploring with index finger at 7½ months.

7½ months
Does he explore the 'Smartie' with index finger before grasping it (Fig. 8.1)?

This occurs normally once in three repeat tests from 7½ months.

Awareness that objects even when out of sight are still there begins from 6½ months of age.

PERMANENCE OF OBJECTS TEST
Material: a woollen or soft plastic ball of not more than 7.5 to 10cm in diameter.

Method: roll the ball across the table between your hands twice, then flick it gently over the outer edge of the table, at not more than 0.5m from the infant.

6½ months: does the infant hold his gaze at the point where the ball disappears over the edge for two to three seconds before looking back at you?

7½ months: does the baby move his head to search the floor for the ball at least once in three successive repeats of the test?

Nine months: does the infant move to search for the ball every time? Failure to search for the ball at 10 months suggests a developmental delay or severe vision problem.

An infant of nine months is expected to explore a small object with the index finger every time before he grasps it using an inferior pincer grasp (*i.e.* uses the first and second fingers at the ends of the phalanges and the thumb). Normally young children experiment with either hand well into the second or third year.

A few infants may use index finger approach with the left hand earlier than with the right. In such cases, mothers when questioned often confirm that there are left-handers in the family or even that she herself had suspected that the infant 'is going to be left-handed'. This is interesting and suggests that dominance for *fine* movements may be determined earlier than previously thought.

10 months: does the infant pick up a small object (such as a Smartie) with a superior pincer grasp? (tip of the index finger and the thumb).

Delay in acquiring this sequence of grasps suggests mental handicap or severe vision defect. If one hand is not used, suspect a motor disorder.

10 to 12 months: infants during this period spontaneously pick up small toys to throw them forward. Repeated practice for three or four weeks leads to the ability to release an object competently from the hand. This can be shown in a combined language/performance test—'Give me' test using a 2.5cm cube (see p. 53). The infant at 10 months offers the cube but takes it back showing that he understands the situation. Two weeks later he presses the cube down in your hand but still takes it back. At 11 months on average he opens his hand and releases the cube into yours.

13 to 20 months: it is wise to seat young children from 13 months upwards at a nursery table. It is a difficult period for developmental examination because the child's attention control is fixed and rigid on one situation or object. Mother's presence is necessary to give him a sense of security, but if too close may promote rejection of a relationship with you.

BUILDING CUBES

A great deal can be learned about the function of the upper limbs at any age from observation of a child building a tower with 2.5cm cubes. It enables you to observe whether the child is right- or left-handed; whether he can use either hand in play; and whether there is any tremor, ataxia, dystonic or other unwanted movements of the upper limbs which suggests a motor problem.

The skill to build emerges from 13 months when a young child acquires finger release and also a capacity to perceive the construction.

METHOD

A set of cubes is scattered on the table. Take up one cube and place it in front of the child; then take up another and give it into the child's hand. Say 'Put it on the top', pointing to the first cube. Repeat the instruction as necessary. Avoid using command words such as 'Build me a tower' which is likely to be incomprehensible to infants from 13 to 18 months of age. 'On the top' is a phrase which together with pointing is likely to be understood.

If the child appears not to understand, show him, then repeat the instruction. Once the child has begun to build, encourage him to continue ('Now another one').

The skill is very variable. The 13- or 14-month-old infant is expected to put up one, but thereafter a wide range of achievement is often seen. It is interesting to speculate to what extent practice may play a part. Bower (1982) reported on the behaviour of identical twins, one of whom had had six weeks' training in stacking cubes, who did no better in terms of speed or number than her twin who had had no training.

Controlled release and an understanding of the task to build a tower of cubes is

Fig. 8.2. Cube models (bridge, train, and three- and four-block steps).

defined as a minimum number of cubes according to age below which, in the absence of a motor deficit, developmental delay should be suspected.

Developmental delay may be suspected if a child builds fewer than three cubes at 18 or 19 months, fewer than five cubes at 24 months, or fewer than eight cubes at 33 months.

30 months to 54 months: while the child is building a tower of cubes you may encourage him to speak to you—an important first hurdle—by saying 'That's a pretty one—what colour is it?' This is a language test in which about a third of children between 30 to 36 months show at least an understanding of the question, often naming one colour for all. All six colours are named on average by 42 months.

COLOUR MATCHING

'Now I'll show you another game'. Take four cubes of different colour, placing them in a well spaced line. Name each colour as you do so. Say: 'Now I am going to find one that is just the same'. Select a red cube from the pool and place it beside its match. Say: 'Now you find me one that is just the same'. This is repeated with several colours.

The graph shows that on average children match colour from 30 to 33 months. Developmental delay is suspected if a child is unable to match colours at 39 months.

COPYING CUBE MODELS (Figs. 8.2, 8.3)

'Now I'll make you something. Shall I make you a bridge?'

Take three cubes and build a bridge behind your hand, out of sight of the child. Then show the child your bridge, and say: 'You make me one like that'. If the child is successful, praise him and tell him, 'Now I'll make you something else'. First sweep down his successful bridge. If you leave his model standing, the 'key' feature of the train, *i.e.* the chimney, will already be in place and invalidate your findings.

Make the train with four cubes behind your hand, before showing it to him. 'You make me a train just like mine'. In order to score, it is essential to perceive the chimney.

The next model, for the child who succeeds in copying the train, is the three-

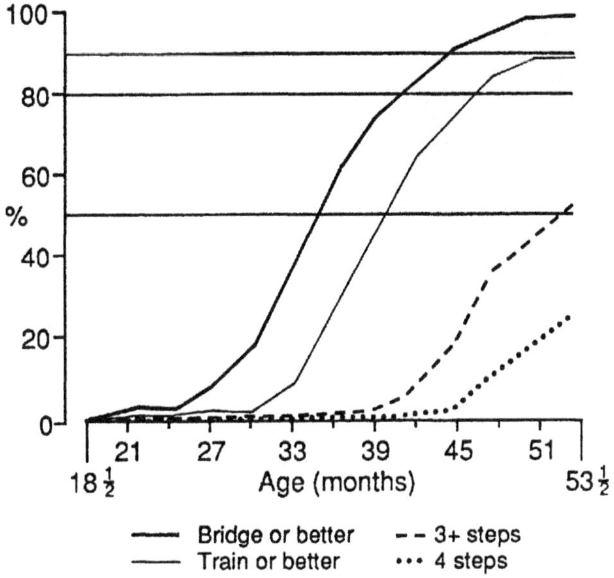

Fig. 8.3. Copying cube models of increasing complexity.

brick steps. The train must be taken down before revealing the new model. 'Make me some steps. See I can walk up my steps', demonstrating the action with two fingers.

RESULTS

50 per cent copy a bridge at 33 months; 80 per cent do so at 39 to 42 months.

50 per cent copy a train at 39 months; 80 per cent do so at 45 to 48 months.

50 per cent copy three-brick steps at 54 months.

Failure to copy a bridge at 42 months or a train at 48 months suggests developmental delay.

COPYING GEOMETRIC SHAPES

Pencil grasp and handedness: place a piece of paper on which vertical and horizontal lines, a circle and a cross have already been drawn down the left-hand margin of the paper. If the child is known to be left-handed the drawing should be on the right-hand margin.

Do not draw these shapes in front of the child. Children are quick to copy your hand movements!

Put the pencil down on the paper so that the child picks it up himself. 'Make me one like this.' Do not gesture the shape, simply point.

Note which hand the child uses. Remember that young children often change hands several times at one sitting. Persistent use of the left hand only suggests left-hand dominance.

Three types of pencil grasp are commonly seen. Children under three years of age may change the grasp several times in as many minutes. The most advanced grasp used should be noted.

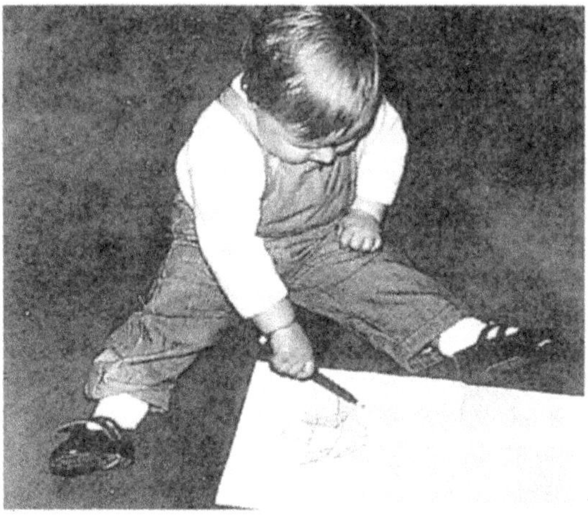

Fig. 8.4. Pronate grasp.

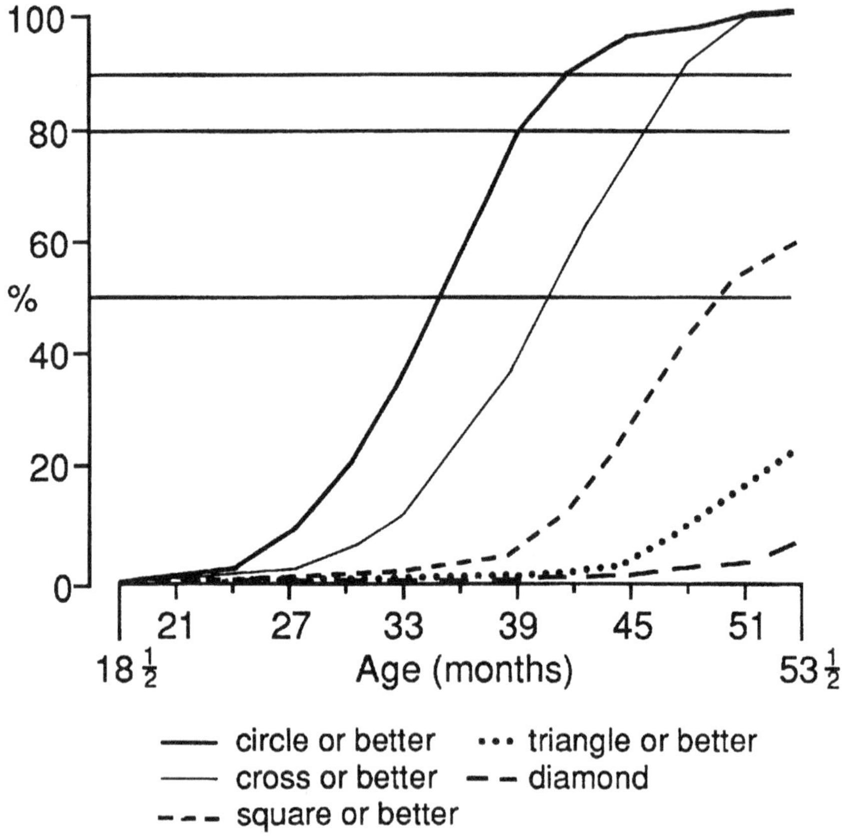

Fig. 8.5. Copying geometric shapes.

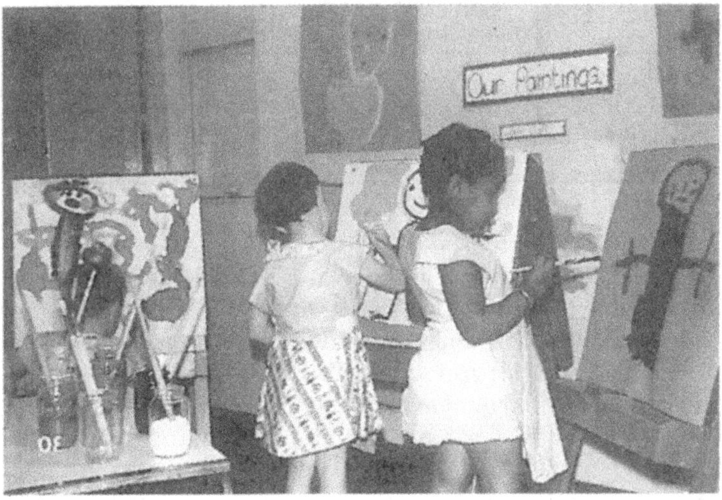

Fig. 8.6. 'Let's draw a man'—4½ years.

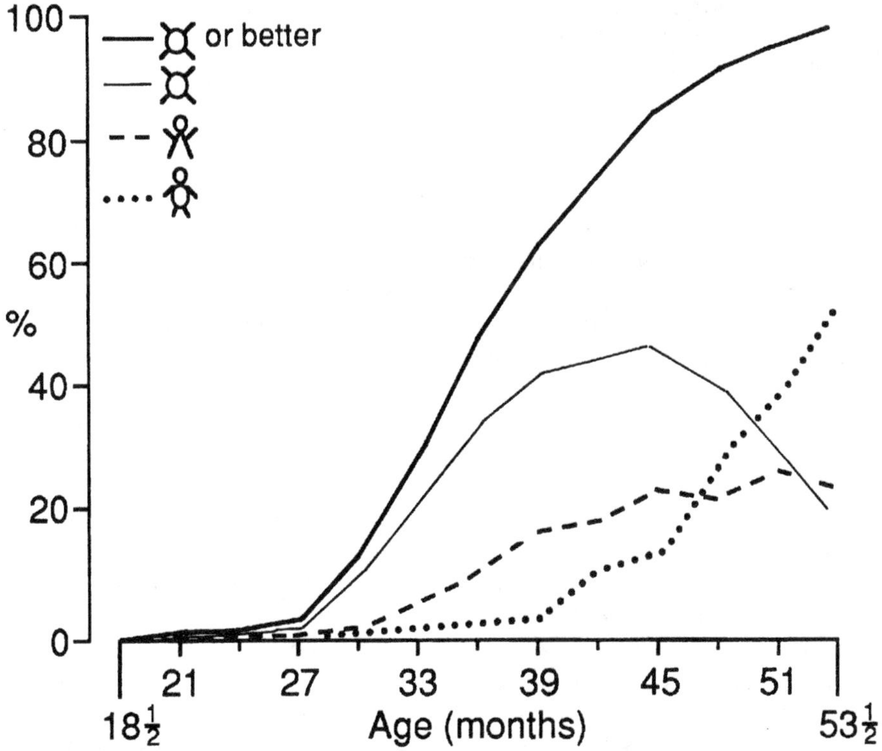

Fig. 8.7. Graph showing draw-a-man test score.

TABLE 8.I
Draw-a-man test

Outline image of human figure	*50%*	*80%*
'Humpty-Dumpty' or better	36 months	42–45 months
Intermediate man or better	48 months	54 months
Mature man	54 months	

The grasps used are (i) *supinate* (pencil grasped at the distal end and often held vertically; present from 18 months but virtually dies out by 36 months); (ii) *pronate* (pencil is grasped in the middle of its length with flexed fingers and thumb (Fig. 8.4); dies out at 42 months); or (iii) *tripod* (pencil held near to the point with thumb, index and middle fingers functioning together. This grasp is used by 50 per cent of children from 36 months. 80 per cent of children have a tripod grasp at 48 months).

Geometric shapes: point to the vertical and then in turn to the horizontal lines, saying 'Make me one like this'. This is intended to encourage the child to begin to draw. Ask him to copy the circle: 'Make me one like this'. Avoid making a circular movement with your finger.

Children on average copy a circle at 33 to 36 months of age; 80 per cent do so at 39 months. Children on average copy a cross at 39 to 42 months; 80 per cent do so at 45 to 48 months (Fig. 8.5).

If a child is unable to copy a circle at 39 months or a cross at 48 months, this suggests developmental delay.

Draw-a-man test

Give the child a plain sheet of paper and a pencil. Say 'Draw me a man—draw Daddy' (Fig. 8.6). Experience suggests that a young child often becomes confused if asked to 'draw Mummy' when she is sitting at his side. The child tends to look at Mummy and back at the paper in obvious puzzlement.

There are three main stages of development in drawing the human figure: (i) 'Humpty-Dumpty' has a head and arms and legs are on the head; (ii) intermediate man, who has a head, no body, legs on head and arms at the right level on the legs. It is not clear that all children necessarily go through this intermediate stage, although some 25 per cent do so; and (iii) mature man, with head, body and limbs on body (p.18).

Goodenough (1926) discerned cognitive elements in the genesis of children's drawings.

The scope of early childhood drawing is universally similar and typical rather than personal (Kellogg 1979) (Fig. 8.6).

The most helpful point of developmental progression is the age-levels at which the three outline images are achieved (Table 8.I).

Developmental delay should be suspected if a child of 42 months is not yet drawing at least a 'Humpty-Dumpty' man, or a child of 54 months is still drawing a 'Humpty-Dumpty' man.

9
DEVELOPMENTAL EXAMINATION OF GROSS MOTOR SKILLS

Walking is a learned skill. Children with severe mental impairment may show delay in learning to walk. On the other hand late walking of itself should not be regarded as evidence of intellectual delay. Age of walking depends on race, culture and family, and may be very variable.

An adverse birth history is important if gross motor disorder is suspected. Family history of shuffling syndrome may be relevant.

A newborn infant in ventral suspension holds spine and limbs in flexion, moves all limbs together and has poor head support. Primitive responses (see p. 3) are present but begin to pass off at three or four months.

The neonate at rest tends to lie for 50 per cent of the time in the asymmetrical tonic neck reflex posture. This is *never* obligatory. If the head is persistently turned to one side, look for constant fisting of the hand on the occipital side. This may suggest a motor disorder. Persistent fisting of the hands after two months of age suggests a developmental problem.

Six weeks

Put the baby in supine on a mattress. Note whether he moves limbs equally and actively. Look for asymmetry of movement.

Head posture

Persistent turning to one side or undue extension suggest a motor disorder. Note size and shape of skull. A rapid increase suggests hydrocephalus.

Pull the baby up to sit (Fig. 9.1). Head lag is expected up to angle of 45 degrees. In upright posture a baby should support head for two or three seconds. Poor head support suggests a serious developmental problem.

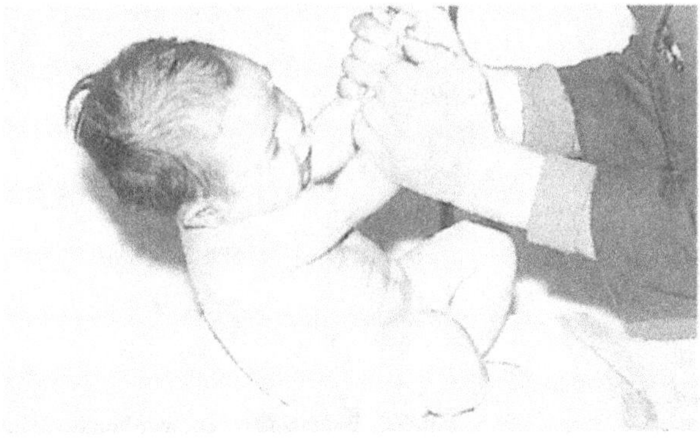

Fig. 9.1. Pull to sit at six weeks.

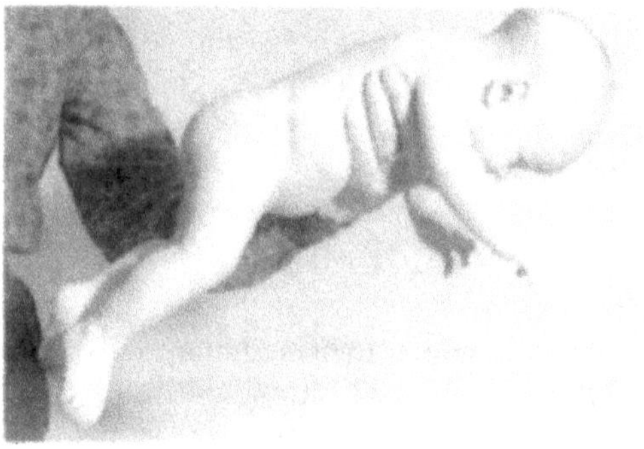

Fig. 9.2. Ventral suspension at six weeks: head in line with back, and some extension of hips.

Ventral suspension

Hold the baby in ventral suspension (Fig. 9.2). His head is held in line with his back, with elbows flexed and knees and hips partly flexed. This is in marked contrast to flexed posture of neonate. Put the baby in prone on a mattress. If the pelvis is high and knees flexed under the body, suspect a motor disorder.

General floppiness should always raise suspicion of a developmental problem.

Ortolani-Barlow test

The hips should always be tested for dislocation. Place baby in supine on a mattress. Hold the thighs and knees flexed with thumbs in front of the thighs and middle fingers over the great trocanter. Fully abduct the thighs and press up on the great trocanter. If the head of the femur is felt to slip into the acetabulum with a jerk, this suggests a developmental abnormality. Repeat on the other side. If an unstable or dislocated femur is suspected, immediate referral for specialist advice is indicated.

16 weeks

Pick up the infant and hold him upright facing the room, then gently tip him sideways off balance (Fig. 9.3). He flexes his head to get his eyes level and at 20 weeks the infant curves his spine to compensate.

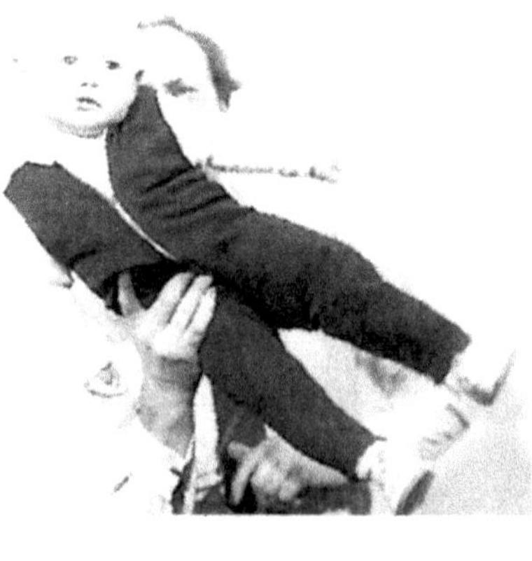

Fig. 9.3. Balancing reactions when tipped off balance at 20 weeks.

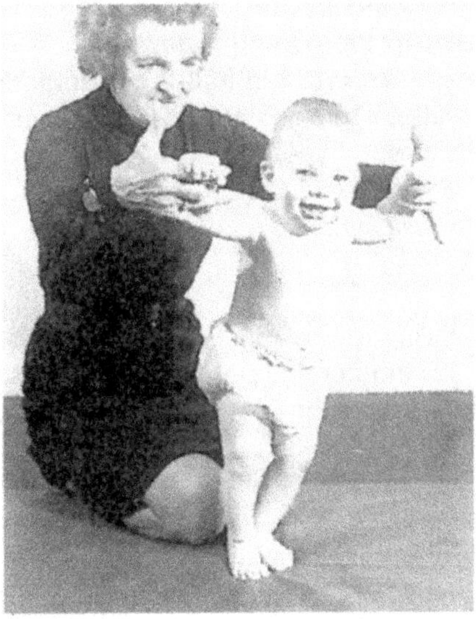

Fig. 9.4. Taking weight on feet with minimum support.

Seven months

Seat the infant on a rug on the floor, with (say) a box of cubes in front of him to hold his interest. Does he sit unsupported? Does he show saving reactions when off balance?

Put him in prone in front of the box of cubes. Does he push up on his extended arms? Perhaps succeed in pushing himself backwards away from the object he wants (eight or nine months)? Does he actually crawl towards it? (10 or 11 months). African babies, especially Nigerians, tend to pass through these stages at an earlier age than is usual in European babies.

Place him in supine. Hold his right leg in extension and with your other hand take his right hand and begin to pull him to sit. Does he try to push up with his left hand on the floor to complete the manoeuvre to sit?

Take each foot in turn by the heel and flex the thigh to a right angle to the trunk to assess muscle tone. Test hips for abduction.

Refer for investigation if there is any abnormality or asymmetry of tone.

Stand the infant upright supported only by holding his hands. He should take his weight on his feet (Fig. 9.4).

Hold child by his hips and tilt rapidly towards the floor. The infant should thrust out his arms in a saving response from seven months onwards.

Remember that children in families with a strong history of shuffling may be a little late in sitting unsupported and somewhat floppy. Follow-up is probably wise if there is an adverse perinatal history.

10 months

Does he sit firmly on the floor and pivot to pick up a toy? Put a toy up to a metre from him. Does he crawl to get it?

Put the toy on the seat of a nursery chair. Steady the chair and observe whether he pulls to stand. Can he lower himself to the ground again?

Does the 12- to 14-month-old step sideways—*i.e.* cruise round the furniture?

Progression to walking and the age of walking are variable within normal limits. Look for failure to take weight on feet, undue hypotonia or hypertonia of limbs, or abnormal postures. *Delay beyond 18 months indicates need for careful examination for possible motor disorder or hip dislocation.*

18 months to four years

Put a toy on the floor and observe the child walking towards it. Encourage him to sit down and play with it. Tell him to take it to his mother and observe if he rises to standing without support. Alternatively he may squat (from 15 months) and rise to standing unaided.

Two years

Play ball, using a soft plastic ball (tennis-ball size). Watch him walking or trotting, bending to retrieve the ball, and throwing it to you. At this age the child generally holds the ball above his head to throw. Encourage the infant to kick the ball. This is variable by age; some boys master the skill very early.

Three years

Observe throw and kick and general movement. Ask him to stand on one foot in imitation of you, then on the other foot.

Four years

The child is expected to be able to hop on either foot.

Abnormality at any age, however, is revealed not by actual milestones of development, but by the pattern of movement.

10
THE MINIATURE TOYS TEST

The miniature toys test was published by Sheridan (1975) to show progressive understanding and creativity of young children in using language codes. The test is widely used by child health doctors for the examination of language development of young children. Ambiguities in the behaviour of children make interpretation difficult.

The test has been modified and standardised (Egan and Brown 1986*b*). Acquisition of expressive verbal labels for miniature household objects and transport; symbolic play shown immediately; and understanding of prepositions were included but not standardised in the original version. Comprehension of questions relating to seven familiar household objects and transport, and a short play situation, have been added.

Standardised data with which to compare an individual child's score are given for all sections.

Purpose of the test

1. Expressive verbal labels for miniature household objects and transport.
2. Symbolic play—self-related and detached-from-self (or doll-orientated) play.
3. Comprehension of questions related to the objects presented.
4. Comprehension of verbal instructions using prepositions.
5. Short play period introduced by a verbal direction.

Equipment

A set of miniature toys—table; chairs (2); cups (2); plates/saucers (2); teapot; bath with taps; jug; aeroplane; sugar bowl; spoon; ship; fork; teapot lid; and knife. All must be miniature size, *e.g.* height of cup 2.5cm, chair 5cm. Second series of toys—undressed doll (5cm); dressed doll; cat; dog; big dog (4cm).

Method

Seat the child at a nursery table. Seat yourself in front with the box of toys concealed from view.

Produce each toy in turn. The order of presentation is: table, two chairs, two cups and saucers, teapot, bath, jug, aeroplane, sugar bowl, spoon, ship, fork, teapot lid, knife.

Expressive verbal labels

As each toy is presented, ask the child 'What is it?' Children on average name four miniature toys at 24 months, eight at 30 months, 12 at 36 months and all at 45 months (Fig. 10.1, Table 10.1).

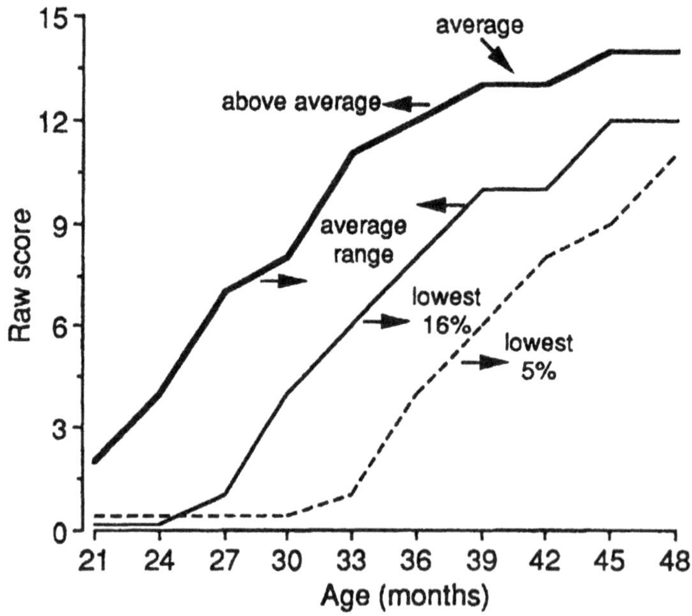

Fig. 10.1. Graph of miniature toys expressive verbal labels score.

Developmental delay is suspected if a child of 24 months cannot name any toys; at 36 months at least six; and all at 51 months.

Symbolic play

Observe the child's action as he takes each toy.

Detached-from-self play	—	appropriately relating one toy to another
Self-related play	—	showing his understanding of its function in relation to himself
Inappropriate play	—	for example, putting the aeroplane in the bath
Indeterminate play	—	putting the toy down without interest defeats interpretation

Children on average at 20 months place the chairs on the miniature table and put the china on the big table in a straight line.

TABLE 10.I

Total score for EVL achieved by at least 50% and 80% of children by age

	Age (months)											
	18	*21*	*24*	*27*	*30*	*33*	*36*	*39*	*42*	*45*	*48*	*51*
50%	0	2	4	7	8	11	12	13	14	14	14	14
80%	0	0	0	2	4	6	9	10	11	12	13	14

Figures refer to the raw score for naming 14 toys used in the test (*i.e.* table, chair, cup, plate, teapot, bath*, jug, aeroplane, sugar-bowl, spoon, ship, fork, teapot lid and knife—raw score 15).
*Scores 2 as questions are posed about the bath and its taps.

Chairs are put correctly to the miniature table and household objects arranged appropriately on average at 30 months. The function of a lid is also recognised but may be put on a cup or sugar bowl instead of the teapot.

Symbolic play with aeroplane and ship are difficult to define. The aeroplane is held up in the air by 30 per cent at 20 months. This gesture then becomes less common. The aeroplane is placed deliberately well away from household objects on average at 42 months. The ship is often placed close to the aeroplane at 42 months, thus categorising transport.

The distinction between self-related and detached-from-self play is clear and sharp yet seems to vary widely. The same child does not necessarily give the same level of play with cup, spoon, jug and teapot. It is difficult to see why there should be this difference with objects that seem so closely related.

Indeterminate play is substantial at all ages and with all household objects. Interpretation is especially difficult with cutlery, which many children tend to 'bunch' in one hand.

Inappropriate action is always significant.

1. Comprehension of questions

Seven questions are asked about the bath, jug, aeroplane, ship, teapot lid, knife, at the time each is given to the child:

Bath — introduce by 'What are these?', pointing to the taps. This is not scored.
Q1. What comes out of the taps?
Q2. Why do we have two taps on the bath?
Jug — Q3. What does Mummy put in the jug?
Plane — Q4. Where do you see aeroplanes?
Ship — Q5. Where do you see ships?
Lid — Q6. Why do we put a lid on the teapot?
Knife — Q7. What does Mummy do with a knife?

Each question is asked when the toy to which it refers is given to the child. There is a very useful developmental gradation in comprehension of these questions which is significant ($p<0.001$).

Level 1

Q4. Where do you see aeroplanes?
Q7. What does Mummy do with a knife?
Q1. What comes out of the taps?

All three questions are understood on average at 30 to 33 months (80 per cent at 39 months).

Level 2

Q5. Where do you see ships?
Q3. What does Mummy put in the jug?

Understood on average at 36 to 39 months (80 per cent at 42 months).

TABLE 10.II

Comprehension of prepositions: responses by 50 and 80 per cent of children

Preposition	*50%*	*80%*
In	21 months	27–30 months
On	24 months	33 months
Under	30–33 months	39 months
Behind	42 months	51 months
In front of	53 months	

Level 3

Q2. Why do we have two taps on the bath?

Q6. Why do we put a lid on the teapot?

Children on average gave correct or sensible answers to both questions at 48 months. This is almost a year later than level 2 questions.

2. Comprehension of prepositions (Table 10.II, Fig. 10.2)
The second series of toys is used in this section.

(1) Put the baby in the bath (undressed doll)
(2) Put the dolly on the chair (dressed doll)
(3) Put the cat under the table
(4) Put the dog behind the chair
(5) Put the big dog in front of the aeroplane

A child's action in (1) and (2) cannot always be distinguished indubitably from merely relating two objects together, because the options are too limited.

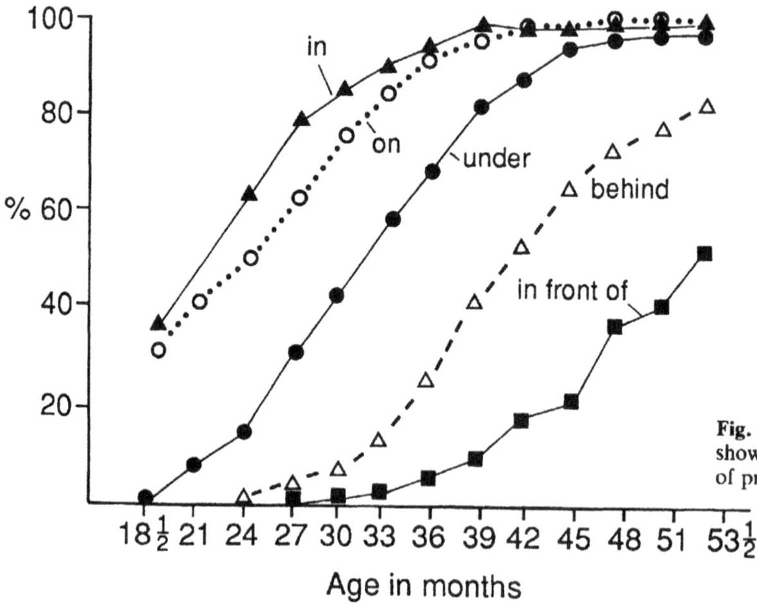

Fig. 10.2. Percentage showing comprehension of prepositions by age.

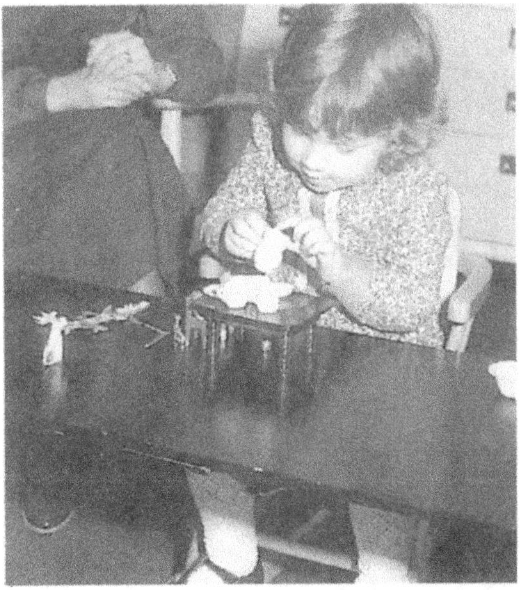

Fig. 10.3. 'Would you like to give Mummy a cup of tea?'

It is interesting that a few young children in the 20 to 30 months age-group placed the doll on the chair on which they themselves were sitting. This is clearly understanding of 'on' related to self.

(3): response is unequivocal.

(4) and (5): action taken to show understanding of 'behind' and 'in front of' is not easily interpreted. In either instance the dog may be correctly placed or if put on the far side of the chair is this 'behind' in relation to the child himself? Similarly is the big dog to be placed in front of the nose of the plane? If placed beside the plane in a position opposite to the child himself, is this 'in front of' in relation to self?

Short play period

When the test for prepositions has been completed, all the toys will be out on the table.

Ask the child, 'Would you like to give Mummy a cup of tea?' (This avoids giving a direct instruction to pour tea.) (Fig. 10.3).

Children in all age-groups on average simply hand a cup to mother. Only a third of children in the 51 months age-group give a sequence of pouring tea from the teapot, adding milk and sugar, or sometimes stirring the tea. If the child does not follow this sequence, ask him 'Would Mummy like some milk in her tea?' (This avoids giving a direct instruction to pour milk.) After this prompt, children carry out a full pretend sequence—pouring from the teapot, adding milk and sugar—at 33 months. 80 per cent do so at 48 months.

The distinctive features of the original test (Sheridan 1975), which was not standardised, were the observation of symbolic play and understanding of prepositions. Responses in these areas are not always clear-cut and require considerable clinical judgement in their interpretation.

The scope of the test is broadened by standardised data relating to expressive verbal labels score, and to developmental sequence by age of a child's understanding of questions relating to the function of miniature household objects and transport.

A significant sex difference in relation to domestic play as shown by serving tea, suggests the material may be more suited to girls than to boys. Lowe (1975) found a similar sex bias.

Conclusion

The test itself is time-consuming, and it requires long experience of the behaviour of young children in this situation. Inherent ambiguities probably make the test less suited to the needs of primary-care doctors and health visitors concerned to reveal a developmental problem. The level of symbolic understanding may, on the other hand, be of great importance to secondary-care paediatricians in the analysis of language disorders and in the planning of intervention programmes for children with severe developmental problems.

BIBLIOGRAPHY

Abercrombie, M. L. J. (1969) 'Eye movements and perceptual development.' *In* Gardiner, P., Mac Keith, R., Smith, V. (Eds.) *Aspects of Developmental and Paediatric Ophthalmology. Clinics in Developmental Medicine, No. 32,* London: S.I.M.P. with Heinemann Medical. pp. 15–24.

Atkinson, J., Braddick, O. J., Durden, K., Watson, P. G., Atkinson, S. (1984) 'Screening for refractive errors in 6–9 month old infants by photorefraction.' *British Journal of Ophthalmology,* **68,** 105–112.

Baird, G., Hall, D. M. B. (1985) 'Developmental paediatrics in primary care: what should we teach?' *British Medical Journal,* **291,** 583–586.

Bax, M., Hart, H., Jenkins, S. M. (1990) *Child Development and Child Health.* Oxford: Blackwell Scientific.

Bower, T. (1982) *Development in Infancy and Childhood, 2nd edn.* San Francisco: W. H. Freeman.

Braddick, O. (1986) *Personal Communication.*

Brown, M. J. K. M., Richards, S. H., Ambegaokar, A. G. (1978) 'Grommets and glue ear: a five-year follow up of a controlled trial.' *Journal of the Royal Society of Medicine,* **71,** 353–356.

Cattell, P. (1960) *Measurement of Intelligence of Infants and Young Children.* New York: Psychological Corporation.

Chaplais, J. de Z., Macfarlane, J. A. (1984) 'A review of 404 "late walkers".' *Archives of Disease in Childhood,* **59,** 512–516.

Cooper, J., Moodley, M., Reynell, J. (1978) *Helping Language Development: a Developmental Programme for Children with Early Language Handicap.* London: E. Arnold. pp. 26–29.

Court, S. D. M. (Chairman) (1976) *Fit for the Future. Report of the Committee on Child Health Services.* London: H.M.S.O.

Davies, B. (1988) *Personal Communication.*

Egan, D. F., Brown, R. (1984*a*) 'Vision testing of young children in the age range 18 months to 4½ years.' *Child: Care, Health and Development,* **10,** 381–390.

—— —— (1984*b*) 'Developmental assessment: 18 months to 4½ years. The bus puzzle test.' *Child: Care, Health and Development,* **10,** 162–179.

—— —— (1986*a*) 'Developmental assessment: 18 months to 4½ years. Performance tests.' *Child: Care, Health and Development,* **12,** 339–349.

—— —— (1986*b*) 'Developmental assessment: 18 months to 4½ years. The miniature toys test.' *Child: Care, Health and Development,* **12,** 167–181.

Francis-Williams, J. (1976) 'Early identification of children likely to have specific learning difficulties: report of a follow-up.' *Developmental Medicine and Child Neurology,* **18,** 71–77.

Fry, J. (1970) 'Acute otitis media in general practice.' *Proceedings of the Royal Society of Medicine,* **63,** 741–742.

Gardiner, P. A. (1982) *The Development of Vision. Studies in Developmental Paediatrics, Vol. 3.* Lancaster: MTP Press.

Goodenough, F. (1926) *Measurement of Intelligence by Drawings.* New York: Harcourt Brace & World.

Hall, D. M. B. (1988) 'Clumsy children.' *British Medical Journal,* **296,** 375–376.

Hamilton, P., Owrid, H. L. (1974) 'Comparison of hearing impairment and of socio-cultural disadvantages in relation to verbal impairment.' *British Journal of Audiology,* **8,** 23–27.

Ikeda, H. (1980) 'Visual acuity, its development and amblyopia.' *Journal of the Royal Society of Medicine,* **73,** 546–555.

Illingworth, R. S. (1970) *Development of the Infant and Young Child: Normal and Abnormal, 4th edn.* Edinburgh: Livingstone.

Ingram, R. M. (1980) 'The possibility of preventing amblyopia.' *Lancet,* **1,** 585–587.

—— Traynar, M. J., Walker, C., Wilson, J. M. (1979) 'Screening for refractive errors at age 1 year: a pilot study.' *British Journal of Ophthalmology,* **63,** 243–250.

Jenkins, S., Owen, C., Bax, M., Hart, H. (1984) 'Continuities of common behaviour problems in preschool children.' *Journal of Child Psychology and Psychiatry,* **25,** 75–89.

Kellogg, R. (1979) *Children's Drawings and Children's Minds.* New York: Mayfield.

Lowe, M. (1975) 'Trends in the development of representational play in infants from one to three years—an observational study.' *Journal of Child Psychology and Psychiatry,* **16,** 33–47.

McCormick, B. (1977) 'The toy discrimination test: an aid for screening the hearing of children above a mental age of two years.' *Public Health,* **91,** 67–73.

Mittler, P. (1972) 'Psychological assessment of language abilities.' *In* Rutter, M., Martin, J. A. M. (Eds.) *The Child with Delayed Speech. Clinics in Developmental Medicine, No. 43.* London: S.I.M.P. with Heinemann Medical; Philadelphia: Lippincott. pp. 106–119.
Moskowitz, B. A. (1978) 'The acquisition of language.' *Scientific American,* **239,** 82–96.
Newsom, E. (1976) 'Parents as resources in diagnosis and assessment.' *Review of Research Practice,* **19,** 105–117.
Piaget, J. (1951) *Play, Dreams and Imitation in Childhood.* London: Heinemann.
Robson, P. (1970) 'Shuffling, hitching, scooting or sliding: some observations in 30 otherwise normal children.' *Developmental Medicine and Child Neurology,* **12,** 608–617.
Rutter, M., Graham, P., Yule, W. (1970) *A Neuropsychiatric Study in Childhood. Clinics in Developmental Medicine, Nos 35/36.* London: S.I.M.P. with Heinemann Medical.
Sheridan, M. D. (1975) *Stycar Hearing Tests.* Windsor: N.F.E.R.
—— (1976) *Stycar Language Test Manual for Symbolic Play Test.* Windsor: N.F.E.R.
Sonksen, P. M. (1979) *Neurological Development and Paediatric Findings Associated with Significant Disabilities of Language Development in Pre-School Children.* M.D. Thesis, University of London.
—— (1985) 'A developmental reappraisal of clinical tests of hearing for normal and handicapped children. Part one: The normal child—principles and the distraction era. Part two: The normal child—the language era and conditioning.' *Maternal and Child Health,* **10,** 122–126, 154–158.
—— Levitt, S., Kitsinger, M. (1984) 'Identification of constraints acting on motor development in young visually disabled children and principles of remediation.' *Child: Care, Health and Development,* **10,** 273–286.
—— Macrae, A. J. (1987) 'Vision for coloured pictures at different acuities: the Sonksen Picture Guide to Visual Function.' *Developmental Medicine and Child Neurology,* **29,** 337–347.
—— Silver, J. (1988) *The Sonksen-Silver Acuity System. Test System and Instruction Manual.* Windsor: Keeler.
Stevenson, J., Richman, N. (1976) 'The prevalence of language delay in a population of three-year-old children and its association with general retardation.' *Developmental Medicine and Child Neurology,* **18,** 431–441.

INDEX